THE PAIN GAME

THE PAIN GAME

C. Norman Shealy, M.D.

CELESTIAL ARTS
Millbrae, California

CELESTIAL ARTS
231 Adrian Road
Millbrae, California 94030

First Printing, April 1976
Made in the United States of America

Library of Congress Cataloging in Publication Data

Shealy, C   Norman, 1932-
    The pain game.

    1. Pain.   2. Pain—Psychological aspects.
3. Biofeedback training.   I. Title.
RC351.S48   616'.047   75-28770
ISBN 0-89087-157-4

    4 5 6 7 — 81 80 79

CONTENTS

ACKNOWLEDGMENTS

Like so many physicians trying to understand patient problems, I am indebted to Eric Berne who taught us that we humans play a series of games as part of our overall life script. Unfortunately, many of the games lead to a loser-take-all stalemate. In no situation is this more true than when chronic pain persists months or years after an unsuccessful attempt at treatment. I became aware of the frustration of managing such patients early in my neurosurgery residency; and in 1963, when I completed my training, I hoped I'd never see another pain patient, for I was convinced then that they were all faking. That's how little psychology I knew! And it also reflects a general medical attitude.

As I entered the practice of neurosurgery, where about one-third of the patients referred are suffering from pain, it became obvious that the primary problem lay not with the patients but with our therapeutic approach (actually physicians are really faking when we pretend to ourselves or to patients that the destruction of nerve tissue is capable of effecting pain relief permanently).

Thus this book is primarily the result of my education by several thousand patients that most pain begins as a simple physical insult. If only we physicians handle the problem appropriately *at the beginning,* the complex personality changes evoked by drugs, surgery and failure would rarely evolve into the Pain Game.

I am indebted to Ron Melzack and Pat Wall for stirring my curiosity with their "gate" theory; to Bill Fordyce for his exciting work in operant conditioning; to Tom Mortimer who built the first dorsal column stimulator (DCS) and worked out the engineering requirements; to Stan McDonald and Norman Hagfors who were largely responsible for the early clinical development of DCS; to Paul Bucy and *Surgical Neurology* for permission to use parts of my papers which have appeared in that publication (these are related to transcutaneous nerve stimulation and dorsal column stimulation); to Sr. Mary Gregory Hanson and Don Kershaw who made possible the development of The Pain Rehabilitation Center concept; to my secretary Kitty Althoff, who has survived over four years of my hectic life script; to Sonja Schrag who has organized and rewritten this book script numerous times; and to my wife and children who have sustained me through the extremes of emotions roused by my part as referee in the Pain Game and who have been left alone while I have tried for four years to spread this message to thousands of listeners. Despite my evangelical approach at times, I emphasize that this is not a religion as indicated by one program chairman who called me the "High Priest of Pain." Every game has a variety of plays and endings. Hopefully the approach discussed here will help more patients choose a winning life-style. Finally, I am greatly indebted to my wife who has significantly helped edit my style.

C. Norman Shealy, M.D.
LaCrosse, Wisconsin

CHAPTER I

Games Patients Play

Most physicians who encounter chronic-pain patients are frustrated both by the patient himself and by the failure of traditionally prescribed treatments. Looking upon these patients as they do alcoholics, physicians often write them off as hopeless cases, beyond medical help. Sensing the doctor's hostility, the patient responds with more of his own. Often expecting some single-handed miraculous cure, the patient goes on his rounds from doctor to doctor in a futile effort to find relief. And far too often the treatment he receives only aggravates his hostility and his pain.

This, in short, is the pain game: an expensive and emotionally debilitating experience for the patient and his family and a long-standing disappointment for the medical profession. The title of this book, *The Pain Game*, suggests transactional analysis. Indeed, the term "game" as we use it refers to the methods of behaving and reacting by the patient, the reactions of his family and even his doctor, which have developed in response to the pain itself. However, our personal approach to the pain game, that is, the learned behavior, is not the same as that of transactional analysis. We are not being cynical when we use the term "pain game" and do not wish to make light of chronic suffering; there is nothing pleasurable or funny about it as the misery of patients and the unhappiness of their families can testify. Furthermore, doctors taking care of these patients usually find very little that is laughable.

On the other hand, as long as the patient allows his suffering to govern his behavior, that is the "game" he is playing, and there is little chance for relief. As the game has traditionally been played, there are no winners.

Pain is more than a hurt; it is to all too many a way of life. Whereas it may begin as a short game, it sometimes becomes a life script. As a symptom it implies a serious or potentially serious disturbance in the body. It is the reaction to pain, however, that determines whether the symptom becomes a habit. The nervous system is a remarkably flexible, plastic mechanism, but it easily adapts to recurrent sensations which can then be just as established as withdrawal from a hot flame.

From the patient's point of view, his therapy has usually been ineffective, sometimes destructive, and very costly. The toll of pain in terms of human suffering and unhappiness is remarkable. There is no way, of course, to price misery. But statistics show that billions of dollars either are expended for medical care payments or are lost to our economy by lowered productivity among pain patients. The average chronic pain patient has had medical and surgical expenses ranging from $50,000 to $100,000. The record in our experience was a man who had had, previously, forty operations with medical costs of $450,000, all originating from an injured back which led eventually through cordotomy, trophic ulcer changes, an amputated limb, phantom limb pain, cingulomotomy, etc.

Statistics defining the costs to business and industry from chronic pain patients are probably conservative, but even at that the following data emphasize the seriousness of the chronic pain problem. Even the most optimistic survey allows that only 39 percent of workmen's compensation patients who have suffered back injuries return to work.

Although the chronic pain sufferers represent a mere 2 or 3 percent of the total number of people injured at work (and they are involved in only 7 percent of the major accidents), somewhere between 50 and 75 percent of the medical costs of workmen's compensation goes for their treatments. What makes matters even worse is that medicine and industry are often helping to create the chronic pain invalid. Knowing how much such workers can cost, employers are often antagonistic to the employee who has had an accident at work, so the patient whose physical condition has already been devastated by injury and the concomitant inactivity is often resented when he returns to work and is given jobs even more difficult than he had prior to his injury. The case of one of our workmen's compensation patients is all too typical.

A 26-year-old manager of a plumbing supply department suffered a dislocated right shoulder after an eight-foot fall. Treated by ʿ general surgeon, he was advised to stay home and "do nothing" for three months; after that time he was told by his doctor that his shoulder was well-healed and that he could simply return to work on the following Monday. On his first day back at work, the man, now twenty-five pounds heavier for all his inactivity, was assigned a so-called light-duty job: painting! Understandably, he barely managed to make it through the first day; complaining of marked shoulder pain, he was told by his employer that since there were no tasks less strenuous than the one he was given, he was out of a job. Unfortunately, most of our workmen's compensation patients tell similar stories. Even if a patient does not like his job (and that feeling may have set him up for an accident in the first place) he is often nevertheless afraid of losing it. His employer's hostility is often more of an emotional strain than he can endure. He is not only out of work for the time being, he is well on his way to becoming a chronic pain invalid. Once he has been off work for two years, it is unlikely that he will ever feel as though he can return to work.

All in all, a patient's personality and his behavior are very much a part of his problem and consequently have to be reckoned with. A very common line among our patients whenever they speak of their pain is "You have to learn to live with it!" Perhaps the patient wants to be applauded for withstanding his suffering (perhaps he should be) but I think this is an indication that his pain has become very much a habit. Some patients build their life-style around their pain, enjoying poor health. Relieving their pain actually disrupts their attitude-behavior system, and neither the patient nor sometimes his family may adjust happily to the change. At the very least, pain behavior is like a mindless bad habit that can be broken; it can also be an addiction.

It is not surprising that a patient who has experienced pain for any length of time should develop a pattern of behavior consistent with those feelings; a lot of human behavior is similarly acquired. Unfortunately, the patterns of pain behavior are very self-destructive. Regardless of the origin of his pain, the patient may discover that there are coincidental, secondary rewards for suffering or that his pain provides a handle with which he can manipulate others. These games may be strong enough to keep him from recovering and he may thus find it worth his while to keep the pain game going.

At one time or another, a certain posture, particular movements, taking drugs may have prevented or alleviated the patient's discomfort. Consequently, he may continue the posture, or the limp, or the drugs, even if such habits no longer have validity. He learns to live with not only the pain, but with the syndrome of reaction to the pain. In fact, many patients will admit that the drugs they are taking for pain are helping very little, but taking medication has become for them as essential as breathing. Or a patient may have found that his pain habits elicit sympathy, feelings of concern, or even approval—rewards he is willing to purchase at the expense of being in pain. A particular facial expression, a moan, that "pained" look may offer a pleasant pay-off since others usually respond with kind words or efforts to help. Some patients are extremely hostile to doctors or members of their families who refuse to react sympathetically to gestures of pain, which points out for the patient that the response has become necessary and expected. Furthermore, the patient may be urged by well-meaning family or friends, or even his doctor, not to overdo; and, as emphasized before, he usually won't to the point that he becomes so physically weakened that he has no choice but to take things easy. Or the patient finds that being in pain wins great approval. He may take a sort of perverse pride in being the most unfortunate, the longest suffering, and his friends may unwittingly encourage him to establish his worth in this way. One of our patients took delight in letting us know that all of her friends kept telling her, "I don't know how you do it." With that kind of reinforcement for withstanding her pain, it will be hard to convince her that suffering is a frightfully high price for a few compliments.

The patient may also find that pain offers him an easy out of situations which he may find unpleasant. Perhaps it keeps him from a job he doesn't like, or it may keep his children and his spouse from making demands upon him, or it may keep him from a normal marital relationship which he would just as soon avoid. Understandably, chronic pain and marriage do not mix. The divorce rate for pain patients is remarkably high, between 60 and 80 percent, indicating that the worse of "for better or worse" does not often include chronic pain.

For one thing, pain often precludes sexual intimacy, and the resulting conflict is greater than many marriages can tolerate. A typical case, which incidentally illustrates various kinds of pain behavior, is that of a forty-five-year-old patient who arrived at the emergency ward without an appointment and on a stretcher. Insisting on immediate treatment for which she would not leave the stretcher, she had in fact been "ill" for eight years and had had six operations on her lumbar spine. Once admitted to our program, she insisted she was in agony and accordingly spent most of her day in bed. Her treatment included withdrawal from a drug to which she was addicted, insertion of a dorsal column stimulator eventually, and two and one-half months of operant conditioning. When she returned home, she felt her pain had been reduced by 50 percent and her activity level increased by 95 percent. She also felt her mental attitude had been improved by 500 percent! I knew she had refused intercourse before admission, so I cautioned her to resume normal sexual activity when she returned home. And so she tried. Unfortunately, her husband who had become obese was no longer responsive. When I saw the woman again, some ten months later, her pain had been reduced even more, at least 70 percent, but by then her husband insisted upon a divorce. Paying her back for earlier refusing him, he had found himself a sympathetic mistress. Indeed, he expressed himself in just these terms: "If this bitch could do it now, she could have done it eight years ago!" Obviously, he felt himself the loser at his wife's pain game and was extremely bitter towards her. While her emotions were devastated, the wife refused to resume her old game plan, realizing wisely that being a stretcher case was too high a price to pay for a husband. They did wind up divorced. Such problems in patients who have had a chronic pattern of behavior for a number of years are not uncommon. The same thing has been noted in markedly obese patients. Sometimes a woman who has been overweight most of her married life suddenly develops an intense desire to be thin and so becomes slim and attractive; her husband then divorces her because he cannot cope with a woman who is sexually attractive to other men!

More commonly, it is the pain patient who wants to even the score with an unsympathetic mate, or one he at least considers so. The most common complaint is, "He won't discuss anything," which many times translates, "He won't let me discuss my pain." Such patients occasionally have rather flagrant affairs while they are hospitalized at The Pain Rehabilitation Center in LaCrosse. Perhaps they need to convince themselves of their own sexual attractiveness, but more likely since they are warned in our orientation lecture that their spouses will probably find out (the center is in a small town and there is always someone who is nosey enough to know and morally indignant enough to tell) the affairs are *intended* to pay back for the hurt of being ignored. Some patients have gotten into such vivid affairs that they have threatened to divorce their original spouses and marry one of the other pain patients. To date, this has not happened; however, two of the chronic pain patients, both of them severely disturbed emotionally, did get married, neither having been married at the time they came here. Their marriage lasted less than a year.

At least one husband has written to find out, "What kind of place are you running up there?" Of course, I didn't have to tell him that the actual affair took place at a local motel. Another husband, finding out about an affair his wife had had while a patient here, set up a manhunt which we feared would lead to homicide, but luckily ended only in a lawsuit for alienation of affection. Maybe it would have helped such husbands if they had realized that the pain game can accommodate a lot of players and that sexual infidelity is one of the ways the game is played.

Interestingly, some patients manage to play both sides of the game at once. We had one thirty-year-old woman who submitted to eight back operations in eight years, yet refused to allow massage by a masseur, which is a routine part of our therapy. She exclaimed, prudishly, "I'll not have a dirty old man massage me!" Nevertheless, three days later, she was spending her nights with one of the male patients at a local motel. Apparently, what she had in mind was a *young* man. Her brazen behavior prompted one delightful patient to comment, "This place is worse than Peyton Place," which invoked visions in my mind of her listening outside every closed door on the hospital floor.

How ludicrous this game can become is seen in the case of a suave forty-year-old man whose wife had him trailed to our center by a private detective. Some time later, he assured me that the infidelity issue had been settled. A few days later, however, he and another patient checked into a local motel only to learn the following day that the motel manager was also the head of the detective agency hired to trail him!

Many patients also manage to play a good game of "My daughter (or son, husband, wife, mother, father, etc.) is killing me." Family disturbances are extremely common sources for the perpetuation of pain, unfaithful spouses and errant children (errant, at least, in the eyes of their parents) being the most frequent cause for emotional crisis. One of our patients, a fifty-year-old woman with incapacitating headaches, finally admitted that her difficulty began when her blonde daughter married a black man. The daughter had been forbidden to return home, ever, or even to return to her hometown, in order to keep the family secret. Only the patient and her husband knew the details of the marriage. Considering how devastating such tension can be, it is little wonder that this woman was in pain. Unfortunately, she had yet to realize that it was not her daughter's marriage, but her reaction to it that was the genesis of her pain; it was she herself and not her daughter who was the cause of her suffering. In order to find permanent relief, she and patients like her have to learn to separate themselves from what they consider intolerable situations involving friends and relatives. Of course, the complaint against a family member may be only one sympton of a pervasive personality discontent. But, in any case, relief from pain is going to require giving up, among others, the game of manipulating and blaming family members.

Of course, the traditional games pointed out by Eric Berne in his excellent book, *Games People Play*—including "Try to cure me, if you can," which is extremely common among pain patients who actually challenge physicians to cure them—are included in the pain patient's repertory.

Patients having been encouraged so often to take things easy, it is extremely difficult to convince patients that physical activity may be increased without physical harm. If he has a strong desire to resume a normal life, however, we can usually convince him that there are no limits except heavy, straining labor.

It is amazing how commonly patients are addicted or habituated to drugs; this has become one of the major behavioral games. A perfect example of this is a sixty-year-old physician who begged me to take him as a patient to withdraw him from narcotics. He gave a thirty-five-year history of being addicted to narcotics which he had begun for severe migraine headaches. He was taking such massive doses each day, they had begun to interfere with his ability to function as a physician. Immediately, upon entering the hospital, he insisted he could only stay a week, even though he agreed over the telephone to stay seven weeks as I had requested because of his extreme addiction. I told him he could go home immediately if he wanted to behave that way, because we could not withdraw someone of his long-standing addiction so quickly. He was a problem from the beginning, although he did practice his temperature biofeedback reasonably well, but he remained around the ward constantly telling patients, "I know a hell of a lot more than that Shealy does. I could treat you a lot better than he does," etc. Why he could treat them so much better than I was treating them, but not take care of himself, was never quite explained. At any rate, after he had been here for about two and one-half weeks and, according to our nurses, was totally withdrawn from drugs, we suddenly found in a pair of rubber overshoes an ampule of injectable narcotics. When approached on this, the patient reported only that, "I didn't really want to get off drugs, I only wanted to reduce them to a level that was tolerable and that I've done. Incidentally, thank you very much for the temperature biofeedback—I haven't had a migraine headache since I've been here and that's the first time in thirty-five years that I've been free of them for such a long period of time." Obviously, this kind of behavior in such an organized, deceitful way is not easily correctable.

We have also had patients who have been easily withdrawn from their narcotics while in the hospital only to go home, immediately contact three or more different physicians, and obtain narcotics from every physican they can convince of their suffering.

Patients play very peculiar games when they go home. In order to avoid false expectations we send all our patients a brochure explaining our program. Even so, one patient sent to his referring physician a vindictive letter in which he made various complaints hoping, I would imagine, to embarrass or discredit our center. His complaints: that medication was increased or decreased "by the doctor's whim to see what reaction the patient has," to the point that some patients who were on relatively little medication were "given enough medication to really zonk them out"; that the program was too time-consuming because "they try every home remedy known to man before getting drastic"; that we overcharged our patients; that "the nerve blocks, X-rays, and general surgical fees will knock your eyes out"; that we used our patients as guinea pigs, subjecting them "to various trials and tribulations" (which in context referred to massage, ice rubs and electrical stimulation); and that "in short, the place is a looney bin." His physician took him quite seriously because we heard shortly thereafter from him:

> I am shocked and dismayed to hear the things that are going on and what my two patients have been subjected to. I in good faith sent them to the clinic under the premise of something truly scientific, new and revolutionary in the treatment of chronic pain. From the sounds of it, Dr. Shealy is evidently grossly misrepresenting himself in his publications and medical communications. It seems to me that no effort is being made in sorting out what is being treated or any particular planned approach. Such things as acupuncture, rhizotomies, coil stimulations to peripheral nerve trunks, cobroxin, all at the same time! No good has come out of such unscientific approaches not to count the numerous unfortunate people who have been subjected to this type of treatment. One of my two patients, although admittedly a high-strung and emotional person was sent up with recurrent but fairly easily controllable left sciatica returned to my office a virtual cripple with a contralateral foot drop and heavy doses of medication.

I might add that the patient mentioned in the letter did not have any weakness when he left the pain center and interestingly one week after he checked out of our center "a virtual cripple" he ran off to do battle with the Indians at Wounded Knee! Of even greater interest, perhaps, is the fact that almost two years later this same patient requested readmission to our center!

And thus the games go on. And on. It is our job to interrupt them.

CHAPTER II

Games Doctors Play

Can doctors play the pain game too? Oh yes, they can, and do! Primed by lavish drug company advertising and "free samples," pressured by too little time for too many patients or by lack of interest, or by too many seemingly unsolvable problems, physicians are at least partly responsible for the public's rampant druggism: drugs to wake one up in the morning or on the road, drugs to lull one to sleep, drugs to prevent pregnancy, to cure headaches, and in plain terms, drugs in response to the patient's insistent, "Do something, Doctor." In frustration, the physician is most likely to prescribe one of the infinite numbers of available tranquilizers, rarely a solution to any problem and a sure ticket to the merry-go-round of many. But, the patient is at least temporarily off the doctor's back, at least the back of *that* doctor. For often, patients with difficult problems will go from physician to physician and each one will play the game, the drug-pain game. Rare is the physician who will try earnestly to come to grips with the patient's problems; the patient may wish to avoid the issue too, or he may simply be unable to identify legitimate causes.

Doctors often unwittingly play the pain game when they admonish the patient, "Take it easy." Instead of progressive exercise, using the body, pushing himself a bit more each day, the patient exerts himself as little as possible, lies around, the body getting stiffer and the pain more painful, while the patient "takes it easy." Druggism and "taking it easy" go hand in hand, filling the waiting rooms of physicians' offices, lining their pockets, and frustrating all concerned.

Surgeons sometimes play a game which can go on in seemingly endless sequence: "if in doubt, cut it out." Or, "a chance to cut is a chance to cure," or more crudely, "the wife's mink-coat operation." While some medical schools teach that surgery is an admission of defeat and should only be viewed as a last resort, not all physicians agree. Some years ago, as I left the operating room, a colleague remarked, "Just another $400 craniotomy, eh!" The idea of removing a brain tumor had never been equated in my mind with cold cash, but other physicians apparently have other ideas. (By the way, he had underestimated the cost of the craniotomy by quite a lot, he might have been sorry to learn.)

Each surgeon must examine his own conscience when deciding upon surgery for a patient; the prospect of financial award should, of course, not be a determining factor in his decision. Since the incidence of surgery is related to the number of surgeons, however, it is possible that surgery is not always necessary as recommended. For instance, *elective* procedures are performed four times as often on Blue Cross-Blue Shield patients as on HMO (pre-paid care) patients. This strongly suggests that not all surgeons operate strictly out of necessity. In England, moreover, many standard operations are done only half as often (in relation to patient population) as in this country. Chances are good that many of the operations for herniated disc are not totally honest miscalculations!

Among internists and other non-surgical specialists, jokes about the money-hungry surgeons have caused a backlash among many physicians to the effect that all surgery is unnecessary, even though it may be lifesaving. Of course, this extreme position has its perils also. Before submitting to surgery, the patient should be certain that his doctor has answered the following questions to the patient's satisfaction:

1. Why is this operation "necessary"?
2. What are the risks of death and complications?
3. What are the risks *without* surgery? Are there alternative courses of treatment which don't involve surgery? What are the chances with those?
4. What are the chances for the surgery doing what it is supposed to do?

Surgery can never be undone. While a surgeon may cite a 75 percent success rate, the remaining 25 percent failures sometimes come out in worse shape after surgery with long-lasting problems that didn't exist before. This is not said to discourage all surgery, but rather to make patients cautious about the perils: the risk of unnecessary surgery in a country prone to such, and the possibility of failure. Patients should also realize that each is an individual; statistics can never reflect accurately the unique reactions, problems, and successes in the face of enormous adversity of the individual person. On the other hand, if you, the patient, have any misgivings about surgery, *don't hurry to submit!* Explore the alternatives; consult another surgeon for another opinion.

This brings us neatly to another game that doctors play: "That other doctor is a quack." Suppose you have pretty much decided on surgery with Doctor A whom you've known a long time; he once removed your ingrown toenail and the results were excellent. This time your gallbladder is the offender and you're wondering if maybe there isn't a way of peaceful coexistence between you and your gallbladder without surgery. Dr. A hasn't been hasty about the scalpel, but diet and various medications have not helped; he is now urging an operation. Naturally you are a little apprehensive about the thought of major surgery, so you decide to consult Doctor B, your best friend's general surgeon. He removed her gallbladder two years ago, and she is certain she feels ten years younger. Dr. B is most cordial as you explain your problem, frankly telling him you want a second opinion. But when you give him your own surgeon's name, he looks down at his desk, then looks hastily at you and explodes, "Why, that doctor is a quack!" Emotions overcome you: hostility, anxiety, disbelief, and even embarrassment. Added to the apprehension over major surgery, you are needlessly overwhelmed, a hapless victim of the game of snide remarks. On the other hand, how should a physician (or should he or she) indicate to a patient that treatment could be more competently handled by another surgeon, (and not necessarily himself)? Physicians *do* see patients who have obviously been mishandled, operated upon needlessly or ineptly, medicated to the point of addiction without good reason. A responsible physician does not like to see the patient undergo more of the same. Perhaps the patient must learn to be a bit of a psychologist for picking up clues on a physician's competence. A wall full of fancy certificates may not be sufficient proof.

A close relative to the game of snide remarks is "I've never even heard of what you're doing" (so it couldn't be very worthwhile, is the implication). For instance, in 1971, four years after I had first implanted successfully a DCS during which time I had given over fifty papers on the subject, I received the following letter from an orthopedist:

> One of my patients recently told me about your quack operation. I have to assume it is quackery, since:
> 1. I never heard of it.
> 2. I never read anything about it.
> 3. None of my neurosurgical colleagues have heard of it.
>   On the other hand, just in case there is anything to your operation, please let me have full details at once, as my wife has chronic back pain and is very much in need of therapy.

Just ten miles from his office, an outstanding professor of neurosurgery had performed more DCS implants than I had!

In fairness to my detractor, however, I must introduce another game that doctors play all too often, "It's new, so I'll try it." The

DCS is a case in point. Although I developed the device, I maintain that the decision to implant one must be made only after careful consideration of many factors. Relatively few pain patients are suitable candidates for the DCS. Unfortunately, some other physicians have rushed headlong to try the new technique without thoroughly understanding the kind of candidate to which the device is most suited, or even exactly how the DCS is implanted. Consequently, I see a number of patients with a DCS whose pain is not lessened. And then they have new pain at the operative site!

The physician is bombarded through advertising and papers with new treatments and drugs every year. Few of these will stand the test of time; the action, technique or design of those that do will most likely need to be improved and modified as the statistics of usage pile up. The doctor who rushes ahead to try as many new gimmicks as possible jeopardizes the health of his patients and his own reputation for competence in the medical community.

Rare is the patient today who hasn't at least once been victimized by the "it's all in your head" game. The physician dismisses the problem he can't or doesn't want to solve with pen and prescription pad: tranquilizers. With so many people on tranquilizers, who knows the true mood of this country? Over the last thirty years, "mood modifiers," as they are sometimes called, have become the panacea of medicine, cashing in on the sugar-coated hard sell of drug company advertising. Valium® alone (touted as a mood reliever) has become the largest selling drug in the world, though it is widely recognized as *causing emotional depression!* Patients who doctor-shop, picking up a number of prescriptions along the way, often take a combination of tranquilizers and pain relievers, with devastating results. Recently, one patient came to our clinic with two bottles of mixed drugs with instructions to "take one every four hours." One of which? I. addition, the patient was taking four other drugs—a total of eight! At some point, a patient juggling such a combination of potent drugs is likely to endanger his life. In addition, drugs are quite unsatisfactory for the relief of chronic pain, and they are no substitute for counseling or psychophysiologic therapy (autogenics).

Closely allied with the "it's all in your head" game is the implication, sometimes spoken quite frankly, "you're too stupid to understand." Trading on this basis, physicians can excuse many of their own failures. They will fail to explain to a patient the risks of surgery or any other therapy, or the alternatives available. Physicians should be sensitive detectives, but they often are not. They fail to pick up clues or they plainly aren't interested. Consequently, they miss the chance to help a patient, dispensing pills or surgery and a big bill while the patient becomes hostile, or hopeless; neither state of mind is very conducive to good health. Patients' favorite physicians are not necessarily those with straight honors in medical school and a host of certificates to boast about, but those who show a genuine concern and interest in the patient as a person, a fellow wayfarer on planet Earth.

Physicians who fail to explain the possible consequences of a surgical procedure may later be haunted by an angry, vengeful patient. Cordotomy patients are only infrequently told of the risk of impotence. Through the rigors of training, the frequent confrontation with death and horrible, indescribable suffering, doctors often take lightly what may to a patient seem very serious. "This won't hurt a bit" will fail to soothe the patient who suddenly feels an unexpected pain. His reaction will be all the greater because of his fear and his unfamiliarity with the procedure. The physician should care enough about the patient to be honest, to have empathy. A doctor who has been a patient sings a different tune. While I had performed many myelograms, no one had ever told me that you can *feel* the weight of the Pantopaque®. When I had a myelogram, however, I learned that this is a heavy, uncomfortable sensation as the Pantopaque® rolls over the nerve roots. I could feel even a minute amount of residual oil though the surgeon was sure he had removed it all. On checking, he found and removed the remaining bit; the unpleasant sensation was gone. I later learned that this sensation is terrifying to patients who are not prepared for it, and consequently they feel great pain.

It reminds me of the frustration of patients who've been told by a surgeon, "you can't hurt; I removed the cause!"

Surely as unfortunate as the game which dismisses the patient and the risks is the one which exaggerates them: "you'll be paralyzed" game. While being honest with patients, physicians needn't depict a panorama of horrors which may terrify the patient to the point of making him a poor surgical candidate. One individual I know was so frightened by his doctor's description of the complications of surgery for removal of his pituitary tumor, that he left the hospital in the middle of the night and headed for psychic surgery in the Philippines. Three years later he remains asymptomatic, so perhaps he did make the right choice!

Patients must be considered individually. A sphenoid ridge meningioma is a slow growing brain tumor. While the risk of surgery to remove one is usually small, it seemed unnecessary to me to subject a 72-year-old woman to the stress of such surgery. Today, eight years later, she is as well as, and no worse off than, she was eight years ago.

A favorite game among physicians does not really involve the patient directly, though it may involve the quality of care that he eventually receives. Physicians are highly competitive individuals, a quality cultivated throughout their medical training. The game certainly doesn't end when one receives the medical school diploma or one of the treasured certificates along the way. Although physicians have trained at well-respected medical schools, and one can assume that some of the prestigious abilities of the teaching staff has been passed along to the students, physicians delight in establishing a "status order." It goes something like this. Physicians who remain at a medical school or are affiliated with one in some way somehow are assumed to be higher on the pecking order than those who have braved the big world and ventured beyond the cloister of the academic. And the G.P. is, of course, at the bottom of the pile. In fact, some of the finest physicians with a well-honed sensitivity to their patients are in private practice or clinics. University status does not of itself guarantee quality or integrity. The point is that sensitive, caring, skilled physicians can be found in many places, urban, rural, academic and elsewhere, as can their less able or less altruistic colleagues. Patients sometimes are repelled by the thought of going to a large university-affiliated hospital. They are afraid they will be treated not as people, but as "guinea pigs," an attitude which has no sounder a basis than the "status order."

Psychiatrists sometimes like to play the game, "after you've cleared up the physical problem, send the patient to me for his emotional one." Such splitting of the mind and body is impossible, as any successful healer knows.

The "nobody will touch me" game sounds as if it is a patient directed one; but in my experience, it is very true. Despite much talk about physicians wanting their patients back from specialists, neurosurgeons, in general, and dolorologists, in extremis, often find it almost impossible to turn continuing care back to local physicians. Patients who have major neurologic deficits, those with intractable pain, those who are failures of traditional medical and surgical therapy, and those with implanted stimulators are all treated as lepers by many physicians. Even dentists fear patients with implanted dorsal column stimulators. Every physician needs to reach a decision concerning each such desperate case, using several consultants if necessary; a planned, consistent approach is then possible. Most of the time it will involve only kind, persistent counseling and encouragement without weekly or monthly experiments with new drugs—or agonizing over possible surgery with each new or continuous complaint. Then perhaps every two or three years, if complaints persist, a reevaluation by a super-specialist with another consistent plan to follow. Physicians need to have confidence themselves in order to convey it to patients, especially to those patients in whom a miracle cure is not possible.

The various popularity contests and ego-building games that doctors play among themselves are, I suppose, harmless. It is those that stand in the way of ethical and sound medical practice which must be decried.

Always on the watch for quackery, the medical profession is quick to dismiss as more of the same any practice which does not quite jibe with the rigid expectations of the "status order." Acupuncture, claims for vitamin cures and the effects of variations in nutrition are among the suspect.

Actually the greatest challenge facing American medicine today is not acupuncture or cancer or atherosclerosis, but a careful and objective evaluation of Western medicine. How is the Hippocratic requirement met, that therapy must, first of all, cause no harm? In evaluating treatments of disease, thought should be given first to those methods which are at least safe. Herb medicines, folk medicines, faith and spiritual healing, electrical and magnetic influences, diet, philosophy, religion, homeopathy, naturopathy, osteopathy all have their adherents and, we must not forget, their successes. The real challenge is to learn the true values of all therapeutic systems, to know our patients well enough to make suggestions that will suit that entity, to use a therapy that is safe and effective.

This book does not intend to offer the last word in pain control; it emphasizes some sound principles of health and suggests ways that patients can help themselves and their physicians to treat problems most effectively. Since it is unlikely that a single factor ever causes a disease, it is equally simplistic to assume that one therapy will be sufficient to remedy the problem, particularly a chronic one. Mind and body must be realigned at the same time to restore health and to maintain it.

CHAPTER III

The Physiology and Anatomy of Pain

Pain is a very subjective sensation. It is commonly recognized that it is more of a psychologically conditioned response to stimulation than it is a specific function. However, thresholds for response which are interpreted as discomfort or pain are reasonably standard; that is, if one applies weighted pins to a part of the body, the range at which normal individuals respond with a feeling of pain is very narrow. The same is true if one applies a rapidly increasing heat or focal electrical stimulation which is graded as painful.

Early in this century, two major theories evolved about the physiological aspects of pain. One of these was called the "specificity theory," in which it was insisted that specific nerve fibers needed to be stimulated or activated (mechanically, electrically, chemically, etc.) for pain to be felt. However, there are too many skin sensations and deep tissue sensations for there to be a separate type of nerve for each sensation. There are, in fact, only four major sensory fiber types, ranging in size from very small to moderate in diameter. Thus, the "pattern theory" of pain

20

evolved which maintained that fiber size was totally immaterial but that the temporal and spatial patterns of stimulation were the deciding factor. This means that some combination of the two theories is more likely to be correct; that is, a lot of the information that comes in over the smallest fibers, named "C," is deemed painful, but not all information by any means that comes in over the "C" fibers is considered painful by some individuals. On the other hand, no information that comes in over the largest, *beta* sensory fibers is considered painful. Normally, there seems to be a balance between the largest and the smallest fibers such that excessive stimulation of the larger *beta* fiber pathways tends to inhibit information coming in over the small "C" fiber pathway thus providing a natural inhibition of pain. On the other hand, if the "C" fibers are excessively stimulated, then they overcome the *beta* fiber inhibition and "open the gate" getting into conscious appreciation of pain. In a number of disease states, some natural, anatomical upset between the largest and the smallest fibers may result: for instance, in patients who have had *herpes zoster,* "shingles," the *beta* fibers are predominantly destroyed, leaving a dominance of "C" fibers so that even normal touching of these fibers is felt as intense pain. Obviously no further damage is being done when the skin is being touched. This particular kind of pain resulting from differential damage to the *beta* fibers with preservation of the greater percentage of "C" fibers is called sometimes the *sensory deprivation pain syndrome.* This means that since even the most delicate sensation of touch has been lost, the patient feels pain rather than touch.

There is also a great deal of difference in the central nervous system reaction to stimulation of *beta* fibers versus "C" fibers. *Beta* fibers tend to have electrical impulses which travel at a much faster rate (60 to 100 meters per second) than the "C" fibers (about one meter per second). Once they enter the spinal cord, *beta* fibers predominantly enter the part of the cord called the dorsal column; this is the only portion of the entire body in which there is a significant anatomical separation of these fibers which normally are mixed both in brain and in peripheral nerves.

The "C" fibers tend to be distributed very diffusely throughout the spinal cord predominantly in the more anterior parts of the cord and, at any rate, outside the dorsal column. When stimulated, *beta* fibers induce a firing of nerve cells within the spinal cord which lasts ordinarily not more than 200 milliseconds; "C" fibers initiate central firing which lasts for many seconds. Similarly, more mechanical stimulation—touch, rubbing, joint movement, and vibration—all elicit firing that lasts no more than 200 milliseconds. A single pinprick elicits a similar firing of central nerve cells. However, stimuli that normally would be considered painful—electrical stimulation of the skin at greater than 40 volts, pinching with a clamp, heat from a hot soldering iron, or injections of painful chemicals such as formaldehyde or water—evoke very prolonged firing which sometimes can go on for many minutes. Such reactions tend to be generalized within the spinal cord and not so specifically related to the anatomical area, where the stimulus originated, as is touch. Also, there are significant regional reactions; for example stimulation of the face causes firing within the spinal cord and down to the low cervical or neck area but not below that, whereas stimulation of any part of an arm or a leg causes generalized widespread firing throughout most of the spinal cord (sensed as pain or discomfort), at least if the stimulus is of a painful nature. Once the electrical impulse enters the spinal cord, the *beta* fiber material travels up the dorsal column, actually stops and changes course, if you will, through a nerve-cell transfer process at small collections of nerve cells at the upper part of the neck, and the nerve fibers then travel on in a crossed fashion to the opposite side of the brain to enter a portion of the thalamus which is one of the big sensory nerve relay stations in the brain. "C" fiber activity is quite diffusely represented throughout the entire spinal cord somewhat more prominently on the side opposite stimulation; that is, it crosses within four spinal segments, or at least about 60 percent of the activity seems to cross. Once it reaches the lower portion of the brain stem, just outside the bottom of the skull, however, the electrical activity from the pain tends to become more restricted primarily to the central area of the nerve tissue, traveling then in the central core throughout the brain stem and projecting rather weakly up to the thalamus. From a research point of view, it is exceedingly difficult to study anything about the appreciation of pain beyond these electrical influences which have been mentioned.

Emotional reactions are not well understood, although we are quite certain that there is a significant stimulation of and interplay in the deep portion of the brain called the *limbic system*. This involves the deepest part of the frontal lobes and the temporal lobes and almost all of the large collections of nerve cells called the diencephalon. Moreover, the same areas contain all aspects of emotions and seem to surround the central brain areas which control autonomic (involuntary) nervous function.

Historically, it may be that pain relief was attempted by counter-stimulation long before any other treatment came along. Acupuncture, which probably works reflexly, and to some extent through the peripheral autonomic nervous system, certainly has been used as one technique for controlling pain for many thousands of years. For at least two thousand years it has been known that electrical shocks (generally, in those days, of a painful nature) could relieve pain of gout and headache, for instance. For some hundreds of years it has been known also that narcotics would relieve pain. However, in the Western world, narcotics came into general use for relief of pain only about one hundred and fifty years ago; about one hundred and twenty-five years ago anesthetic agents of a more generalized nature became available. The most rapid progress in pain relief has come in this century. Somewhat toward the end of the nineteenth century and the early part of this century, it was demonstrated by many scientists, physicians, etc., that external non-painful electrical sensations, interpreted as tingling, buzzing, vibrating, etc., were capable of relieving pain. Then, in the first quarter of this century, it was demonstrated that one could relieve pain in one leg, for instance, by cutting the opposite anterior half of the spinal cord. This procedure, called *cordotomy*, was widely used for a number of years, but it had significant disadvantages. It quickly became obvious that about 10 percent or more of patients developed paralysis of the leg on the same side on which the cut was made in the spinal cord, although total paralysis was uncommon. Similarly, many patients in about the same percentage developed bladder and bowel paralysis, and sexual impotency complications were not commonly discussed prior to this surgical or knife-type cordotomy.

If the procedure was carried out up at the top of the spinal cord, at about the second cervical area, breathing was sometimes interfered with. If the procedure was carried out on both sides of the spinal cord, many patients developed difficulty breathing; bladder paralysis and sexual impotency were noted almost invariably in that situation. The most disappointing factor in surgical cordotomy was that, while pain relief occurred in about 80 percent of patients at the time of the surgery, it was often short-lived. By the end of a year over 50 percent of the patients, if they had survived their primary disease, had a return of pain. Thus, because of the various complications of the major surgery involved, cordotomy gradually fell into rather generalized disuse, except for cancer pain if the patient was felt to have a life expectancy of greater than three months. About ten years ago, a Chicago professor of neurosurgery devised a technique for performing cordotomy without an open surgical procedure. This was eventually refined into using a radio-frequency heating current applied into the spinal cord through a needle. A great revival of cordotomy ensued and many thousands of patients had the anterior quadrant of the spinal cord burned, cooked, or coagulated, as you prefer. However, even though technically the operation became easier, in my opinion, the results have been poorer.

In fact, a problem seen in surgical cordotomy, post-cordotomy dysethesia, has seemed more common. More about that in a moment. The incidence of paralysis, bladder paralysis, etc. has remained about 10 percent. In my own experience, I have seen only one patient who denied impotency after a unilateral, one-sided, cordotomy done with this needle. Even in that patient, he quite embarrassedly admitted that his potency was diminished significantly. In every other patient I have seen, male or female, the patient has complained that he has been totally unable to have satisfactory sexual relations and in a woman this means no orgasm. In about 10 percent of patients who have undergone the percutaneous cordotomy, there is development of intense, burning, creepy-crawly pain that is nerve-wracking and tends to drive the patients almost insane; this generally involves the arm and leg. Invariably, the patients feel that this intense pain is infinitely worse than the pain for which the cordotomy was done. The treatment for this is extremely inadequate and poor. This is another of the sensory deprivation pain syndromes.

Also, early in this century, neurosurgeons began cutting the entire posterior sensory nerve root in the spinal cord. This has been done at all levels of the spinal cord. It requires a laminectomy, which is a major operative procedure, carries a small risk of two to five percent of paralysis because of interference with the blood supply to the spinal cord, but its greatest problem is that the overall success rate is less than 40 percent. Its lowest success rate, which brings it well down into the under-20 percent level, is in the pain affecting the leg in the so-called low back or lumbar disc syndrome. Indeed, the only place that cutting of a major nerve root has been reasonably successful in relieving pain is in the face where destroying the fifth cranial nerve behind the ganglion, the transmittal center for the nerve at the base of the skull, has been reasonably successful in about 75 percent of cases in relieving *tic douloureux*.

Various destructive procedures have been tried in other parts of the spinal cord. Splitting the spinal cord to try to prevent the "C" fibers from crossing (commissurotomy) has been singularly unsuccessful except in some cases of deep rectal or vaginal pain and has a significant risk of paralysis. Various lesions have been made in parts of the brain stem; these carry a high risk of neurologic complication, i.e. paralysis, and very little chance of long-lasting pain relief. Similarly, destructive lesions have been made in various parts of the brain, including the thalamus with little chance of success in relieving pain. Back about thirty years ago, there was a wide rash of destructive brain procedures done on the frontal lobes; this destroyed the patient's personality almost entirely, but it was noted that they did not complain of pain.

A "refined" (and I use the word loosely) procedure called cingulumotomy has been devised; and for about twenty years has been done in selected cases in which the pain is considered a "depressive equivalent." In my own experience it still has been a frustrating procedure because the patients have a rather blah, bland affect, but continue whining and complaining of pain and are not amenable to either electrical stimulation, behavioral modification or autogenic training.

Thus, in summary, I think we can say that the destructive nerve or nerve pathway procedures as techniques for relief of pain have been largely unsuccessful and fraught with multiple complications. They should be undertaken only in *tic douloureux,* and in patients with cancer pain, and, of course, only as a last resort in any of these situations. They are not procedures which should be undertaken in patients who have "benign" pain, that cause of pain which is not going to be fatal.

Always, if possible, one should try to get at the cause of pain; that is, if there is pressure on a nerve, then the pressure should be removed. This indeed seems to be a rather rare cause of pain and except in certain tumors probably is extremely uncommon. In the last half century, there has been a marked increase in attempts to correct back and leg pain and sometimes neck and arm pain by operating upon discs, the little ball-bearing, cartilaginous-like material which seems to hold the vertebral bodies apart and allow movement. Bits of this material do indeed rupture through their restraining ligaments and press on nerve roots, but, much more commonly, these little bits of disc material just bulge slightly, and cause the joints to collapse somewhat. Pain occurs as a result of disturbance of the alignment of the joints rather than through direct nerve root pressure. When nerve root pressure is not caused by the bulging or degenerative disc, then obviously operating on the disc and removing the bulge is not going to relieve the pain.

CHAPTER IV

A New Way of Handling Pain

In 1965, shortly after Melzack and Wall introduced their theory on the gate control of pain, it seemed to me that someone could best control pain by applying electrical stimulation to the dorsal column (in the backbone) where the *beta* fibers were separated from the "C" fibers. Our research then led to the development of dorsal column stimulation, with the first patient implanted in April 1967. By 1969, I had done only six patients in the early part of the year, and eight patients by the fall of that year; however, a number of neurosurgeons were becoming increasingly interested in the use of dorsal column stimulation for the control of pain. Thus, the dorsal column study group was formed. We invited those physicians who had expressed an interest in the technique as well as a number of neurosurgeons who were prominent in the field of pain. Most of them joined the dorsal column study group except that Dr. William H. Sweet and Dr. Blaine Nashold preferred to do the procedure but not be part of a cooperative study. Increasingly, my own practice became dominated by chronic pain patients who were referred to me in large numbers.

27

Even though I was still doing a generous amount of general neurosurgery, it was obvious I was not handling the chronic pain patient very well. I was selecting about six per cent of the patients who came to me for implantation of dorsal column stimulation; I had nothing to offer the other 94 percent and sent them away. Thus, by late 1970, I realized that there was an intense need for some therapeutic approach to chronic pain that we did not have. And I began to look at the pattern of pain clinics throughout the country.

Largely, because of the work with cordotomy and rhizotomy, neurosurgeons for the past half century have been considered the court of last resort for referral of chronic pain patients. For the purposes of this discussion, chronic pain will be considered that pain which persists six months or more following primary therapy for the disease process causing the pain. It will further be assumed that the primary disease process itself is no longer correctable or curable and that pain relief is the only possible approach to the patient's complaints.

For many years, most of the university centers and many of the major medical centers have had pain clinics. Almost invariably these are considered multidisciplinary; however, in general, this has implied that a patient is screened by one physician who may be an anesthesiologist, a neurologist, a neurosurgeon, an orthopedist, etc. Once the diagnosis is relatively certain, the patient is often then offered the possibility of either psychotherapy, drugs or some consideration for a destructive neurosurgical procedure. Thus, many of the pain clinics predominantly serve as screening clinics for destructive neurosurgical procedures. Nerve blocks are prominently done at clinics such as these and patients are elaborately re-evaluated for the possibility of some further surgical approach.

This whole concept implies that pain is either removable or that the nerve pathways subserving the pain are removable. Actually, there would have been no need to develop dorsal column stimulation or external electrical stimulation, or to consider the possibility of some alternative mode of therapy for chronic pain patients had the traditional destructive procedures been of value in benign pain.

Since the time of my neurosurgical residency, it has been obvious that chronic benign pain, that is non-cancerous pain, should not be treated by cordotomy, rhizotomy, or cingulumotomy as these procedures do not give lasting relief and the complication rate is much too great to be allowable.

Thus, by 1971 it had seemed necessary that we develop an alternative mode of therapy for patients with chronic benign pain. About that time, we learned of Dr. Wilbert Fordyce's work with operant conditioning in the management of chronic pain patients. Although commonly considered a part of the Seattle Pain Clinic, Dr. Fordyce's behavioral modification or operant control program is actually quite separate, and only 25 percent of his patients have come through the pain clinic itself. Overall, also, of all the patients that he personally screens in consideration for the program, only 25 percent are admitted to the operant conditioning program. I was quite impressed with his results in a limited series of 100 patients treated over a five-year period. Sixty percent of the patients with an eight-week operant conditioning program with no surgical or mechanical therapy intervention of any sort were markedly improved, off drugs, etc. However, only an average of about one-third of the original 100 patients maintained pain relief. It, therefore, seemed to me that one could combine the operant conditioning program with the rather extensive mechanical therapy available for control of pain.

As might be expected, my neurosurgical colleagues were not encouraging at the concept of a neurosurgeon giving up his active surgical practice and restricting himself only to chronic pain. However, we knew from a number of surveys that the average neurosurgeon actually has about one-third of his practice composed of pain patients. Therefore, the volume of such work is apparent and it would appear that one neurosurgeon in three could theoretically restrict himself if he had something adequate to offer these patients. I don't believe that would be quite true when we consider the rather huge number of neurosurgeons!

At any rate, in the fall of 1971, the Pain Rehabilitation Center® was opened in LaCrosse, Wisconsin. This facility consisted of a twenty-four bed unit exclusively restricted to chronic pain patients on one of the floors of a local hospital.

Nurses were taught not to pamper the patients or to show any sympathy whatsoever toward their pain. Furthermore, they were encouraged to urge the patients into the various physical activities which had been ordered for them and not to allow the patients to refuse any therapeutic order.

Some immediate modifications were made in the operant conditioning aspect of Fordyce's program. For instance, patients were screened elaborately when they came into the office. We determined first that there was no physical abnormality that was capable of relief. After examination and the patient's history, we arbitrarily assigned the patient a certain amount of walking to do which would vary from about one-half of a city block up to five city blocks per day using the length of the floor as one-half city block. They were further required to ride either a regular stationary bike or a movable, electric bicycle for anywhere from one minute four times a day up to fifteen minutes four times a day. All patients were also required to go to the swimming pool at the YM-YWCA five days a week for a one hour program of swimnastics, an excellent water calisthenics program. The physical exercise was rounded out by limbering exercises which were carried out twice a day, the patients being instructed and supervised by an occupational therapist. Thus, a physical exercise program required anywhere from two to three hours a day with generous rest periods.

All patients were also instructed to use an external stimulator again with much help from the nursing staff as many hours a day as possible. (More about the actual application of the external stimulation will be given in a later chapter.)

Patients' drugs were disguised from the beginning. Initially, we tried disguising each of the patient's drugs. The pharmacist at the hospital refused to mix all the drugs together in a liquid matrix as is done at the Seattle Center. Thus, very quickly, because the

patients objected rather vigorously with nausea and some vomit-
ing to a large number of drugs each separately disguised in a
liquid matrix, we went to a capsule program. Gradually, however, all patients were withdrawn from their pain- and mood-
altering drugs.

Each day the patient was given a vigorous slapping and
kneading massage by a nurse or aide to the area of pain, followed
by an ice rubdown with a frozen popsicle prepared by inserting a
tongue blade into a paper cup of water. Later in the program, an
excellent external vibrator was added to be used on the patient's
entire body once a day and very shortly after the beginning of the
program, a masseur was hired full time to give each patient a total
body massage every day.

The physician consulted with each patient individually once or
twice a week, at which time acupuncture or percutaneous electrical stimulation might be tried. The rest of the week physicians
only checked with the nurses to see if there were any medical
problems that needed to be handled in each patient.

For the first year of the program, a psychiatrist saw each
patient in consultation and group psychotherapy sessions for one
hour three times a week. These proved singularly unhelpful and
exquisitely unpopular with the patients, so after one year they
were discontinued. All patients were given a pain questionnaire
and the MMPI test to evaluate their personalities (see Appendix).

Initially, we thought that each patient might have to stay eight
weeks following the precedent set at the Seattle Clinic program.
However, patients became very distressed at being away from
home quite that long; the first year of the program the patients
averaged thirty-two days each in the hospital. A variety of
possible admitting and discharge procedures was tried. For about
one-half of the time patients were admitted at a rate of six to eight
each week, but this proved to cause a great number of problems;
occasionally a very negative and hostile chronic pain patient who
had been around the program for three weeks would sour new-
comers to the program. Thus, the preferred and much more
successful way of managing the program was to admit all

twenty-four patients within a two-day period and discharge all the patients at the same time.

Initially after the first two weeks, each patient's pain status was evaluated. If pain relief was insufficient, we would then consider the possibility of either dorsal column stimulation, peripheral nerve implantation of an electronic stimulator, or a facet rhizotomy. No other surgical procedures were entertained as possibilities.

The surgical procedure was usually done during the third week of hospitalization and the patient was ready to go home by the end of the fourth week. Patients who were progressing satisfactorily with the external electrical stimulator, operant conditioning and physical exercise program were similarly continued through the program for four to four and one-half weeks.

By the end of the first year of this program, it was obvious that we had not been doing enough to give the patients an adequate program to maintain them at home. We had many more backsliders than we would have liked. To counter this situation, we introduced autogenic training, very shortly thereafter supplemented by biofeedback. Initially, we used biofeedback one hour a day and autogenic training twenty minutes twice a day. This proved extremely inadequate and gradually the amount of autogenic training was markedly increased until the patients were given a total of approximately sixty hours of autogenic training during their course. By the time this had evolved, the entire program had been modified to a three-week program with all the patients admitted on a Monday and Tuesday and all discharged the third Friday. Actually, then, the patients were in the program either eighteen or nineteen days, the only difference from the program as outlined earlier being a very intense use of autogenic training with moderate use of biofeedback supplementation.

In the summer of 1974 we converted to an outpatient program, doing the entire therapy in our office. Only medically ill or seriously drug-addicted patients were admitted to the hospital which is physically attached to our office building. An excellent, inexpensive motel is available in the same building. Patients are treated with acupuncture, biofeedback and autogenic training (at least four hours a day), massage, ice, external electrical stimulation, physical exercise and counseling. The twelve-day program has been quite as effective as the in-hospital approach. Considering the success of surgi-centers it appears that many therapeutic approaches could be converted to outpatient care, if insurance carriers would agree.

Insurance carriers who publicize themselves as doing such a great job for the coverage of medical expenses are notoriously poor when it comes to any form of rehabilitation. We have found that only 65 percent of physicians' bills are covered by insurance companies and even then it is very time-consuming because of the numerous inquiries from insurance companies about the program. About 85 percent of the hospital bill, however, is covered by third-party carriers. These figures must also be tempered somewhat by the fact that about 50 percent of the patients are workmen's compensation patients who have prior authorization to enter the program. Thus the non-workmen's compensation patient is likely to have his physician's expenses paid only about a third of the time and the hospital expenses paid about two-thirds of the time. This leads to a tremendous problem in bill-collecting from non-compensation type patients as patients are accustomed to having their medical insurance cover their medical expenses. Most policies do not cover any form of rehabilitation, much physiotherapy, or any of the mechanical devices, such as external stimulators, which patients may need for continuing their progam at home. Furthermore, when the patients are treated on an outpatient basis, third-party carriers are even more likely to refuse payment of the expenses and as in so many other illnesses this leads to excessive use of hospitalization. I believe that about 50 percent of patients who are hospitalized throughout this country do not need to be hospitalized, but are there in order to have their expenses covered by the insurance company, and obviously this markedly increases medical expenses. Indeed, in a few cases, even workmen's compensation carriers insist that the patient must be hospitalized in order to be treated. This raises the cost of the patient's therapy by about 50 percent and seems totally unreasonable.

Finally, it seems most appropriate to mention that our goals in treating the chronic pain patient are aimed primarily at:

1. Getting the patient off drugs so that he can think straight.
2. Increasing the patient's physical activity to as near normal as possible. This does not necessarily imply the possibility of heavy work.
3. Improving the patient's mood so that he feels happy and reasonably well-adjusted; then and only then,
4. Getting him to return to work.

In our experience, not more than 30 percent of the chronic pain patients who have been disabled two years or more—and most of them have—can be expected to return to work. On the other hand, 80 percent of them are potentially rehabilitatable in the first three categories that I outlined and this seems a very worthwhile goal when we consider the finances of pain.

Fordyce has estimated that his program of operant conditioning lasting eight weeks costing $5,000 in 1971 was financially a break-even situation for society if he could rehabilitate one patient in ten. Since, in the long run, he was rehabilitating about one patient in three, this made his program very worthwhile. The program in LaCrosse initially cost about $3,500 counting all hospital and physican fees. Today, this program if it were still being carried out in that way would cost about $5,000.

The twelve-day program counting the patient's staying in a motel facility and meals, all the medical therapy, etc. averages about $1,500. If we have a success rate of 30 percent for return to work and 60 to 80 percent for getting the patient off drugs and out of the pain-game process, we are doing a tremendous job in saving society money. This I believe is the primary goal at the pain control center. At this point, it appears that 64 percent of our patients remain good or excellent six months later. However, only about 25 to 30 percent can be expected to return to work.

CHAPTER V

Operant Conditioning:
New Rules for the Pain Game

There are certain aspects of pain control that the patient himself must implement: We are, in effect, saying to him, "It's your move!" And, for his sake, we hope he makes it a good one, since his goal of achieving pain relief rests as much on what he does for himself as on what we can do for him.

To that end, we ask that he understand some of the psychological impacts of pain and what it has done to his personality (and vice versa); and we ask too that he agree to change his habits, the way he reacts to pain, and the way he has encouraged, even demanded, that others react to him because of his pain. All of this involves coming to terms with his attitudes and his emotions.

For the pain patient, personality alterations are, in part, the result of his suffering; it is hard to imagine anyone who has been in anguish for any period of time maintaining a normally cheerful, optimistic attitude. Personality changes may also be alcohol or drug induced; considering that some pain patients who have sought relief in alcohol or drugs are literally addicted, personality erosion is not unlikely.

35

But the converse is also true: The patient's pain is probably aggravated and possibly generated by a gamut of negative feelings of hostility, guilt, fear, anger, and frustration. In this way, the pain and the personality problems are self-perpetuating. For purposes of pain relief, however, it doesn't really matter whether the patient's emotional difficulties are the cause or the result of his pain. Either way, as long as emotional conflicts remain unresolved, all physical attempts at pain therapy are likely to fail outright, or if they do succeed, they will often be short-lived successes. Realizing this, in 1971, I restricted my practice to dolorology: the treatment of all aspects—including the behavioral and emotional—of the pain syndrome. My major emphasis since then has been on behavioral modification, also known as operant conditioning, on autogenics or autogenic training, and on biofeedback.

Operant conditioning is simply an effort to encourage the patient to function normally despite his pain. Since it won't hurt him any *more* if he is active, he is encouraged to exercise and begin living a normal life again. Drugs are systematically withdrawn and pain behavior, the patient's pain game, is not reinforced; it is, in fact, strongly discouraged. Autogenics and biofeedback, which will be discussed in more detail later, are methods of achieving self-regulation of the autonomic nervous system. For the pain patient, that means, first and foremost, gaining freedom from his pain; but even more important than he may realize at first, it means that he may be able to maintain, in general, better mental and physical health.

It is almost impossible to be certain which came first: the depressed, angry, hypochondriacal, hysterical personality or the physical illness causing pain which, being unrelieved, led to these traits. Whatever came first, the personality traits of depression, hypochondriasis, and hysteria are so common as to be almost universal among patients who have chronic pain problems which have failed to respond to multiple therapy attempts. Often paranoia and hostility are also part of that emotional profile—as any doctor who deals with pain patients can testify!

Many other clinicians have been concerned with the correlations between pain and personality, realizing that the two are inextricably involved in the pain syndrome. For the past eight years, we have depended upon the Minnesota Multiphasic Personality Inventory (MMPI) and have found it as useful as anything else in determining the extent of our patients' personality problems, information which we have found helpful in deciding which patients are likely to profit from our program; if a patient is severely emotionally disturbed, the chances are not good that treatment will relieve his pain.

Through some 500 questions, the MMPI evaluates personality and reports it in terms of the following traits:

Scale 1 - Hypochondriasis (indicating excessive concern about health and body functions)

Scale 2 - Depression (showing mood fluctuations, worry and pessimism)

Scale 3 - Hysteria (measuring immaturity, repression, and susceptibility to suggestion)

Scale 4 - Psychopathic Deviate (high scores indicate an impulsive personality and low scores a conforming one)

Scale 5 - Masculinity-Femininity (high scores suggesting in females masculine attitudes and in males feminine attitudes and interests)

Scale 6 - Paranoia (indicating suspicious, overly sensitive personality)

Scale 7 - Psychoasthenia (measuring phobias, obsessions and compulsions)

Scale 8 - Schizophrenia (high scores suggesting unusual thought processes and nonconformity; low scores, a conventional personality and compliance)

Scale 9 - Hypomania (measuring the level of emotional excitement)

Scale 10 - Social Introversion (high scores indicating a shy, sensitive personality, a sociable personality)

The MMPI report for the chronic pain patient typically looks like this:

MMPI PROFILE

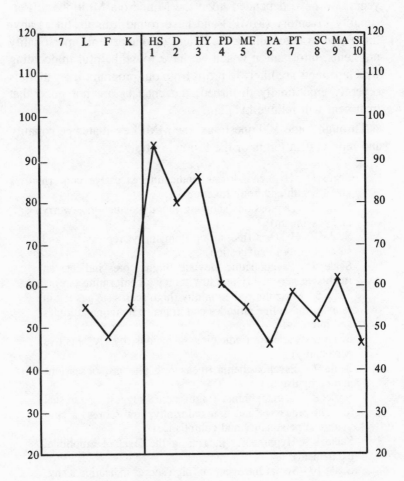

The "normal" range is from 30 to 70 (that is, within two standard deviations from the mean of 50). Only 3 percent of the general population falls outside these ranges, whereas about 95 percent of chronic patients fall outside the range of "normal" on one or more scores. Indeed about 75 percent of our patients have elevations of two or three standard deviations on the hysteria, hypochondriasis and depression scales. A small percentage have elevations on other traits, most commonly paranoia and/or schizophrenia. A recent study analyzing the MMPI scores of 119 chronic pain patients indicates what the authors call "an interpersonal alienation and manipulativeness factor": the tendency of chronic pain patients to place responsibility and blame for their difficulties onto someone else, their feelings of being helpless and different from others, and their need to influence other people. This, the authors point out, offers further support to the point that successful pain control requires the rehabilitation of the *whole* patient; and the test data also verifies the game-playing aspects of pain behavior which are so evident clinically.

Another study, which relied on both biographical data and psychological testing, points out still another feature of the chronic pain profile: the denial and repression of emotional problems. Most patients tested would not admit to conflicts with family members or to difficulties with their jobs; and they also noticeably avoided any reference to unpleasant feelings.

In treating chronic pain patients, the MMPI is of great value in picking out those severely disturbed patients with four to eight personality traits beyond the two-standard-deviation level; they are dangerous, law-suit prone individuals who are almost impossible to help. On the other hand, elevations on the first three traits (hysteria, hypochondriasis, and depression) are common and of no significance in precluding very successful pain therapy. Interestingly, we have not seen scores below 30, indeed rarely below 40, on any scale in the over one thousand patients we have evaluated with the MMPI. *And very interesting too is the fact that once pain control is achieved, the MMPI scores for most patients return to normal.*

In an attempt to determine whether a different set of questions oriented to the pain patient might be valuable, we have used a special pain questionnaire for over three years. (See Appendix for the complete questionnaire.)

After evaluating the questionnaires of four hundred patients and comparing their answers with their MMPI scores and the physician's opinion of their emotional state, only twenty of the questions were found to show significant value in classifying patients as "normal," "slightly disturbed," and "severely disturbed." These questions are:

7. Previous psychiatric evaluation?
   a. yes
   b. no

8. Previous psychiatric treatment for greater than 1 month?
   a. yes
   b. no

11. Have you ever desired it?
    a. yes
    b. no

15. Length of time you've had pain.
    a. less than 1 year
    b. less than 2 years
    c. less than 5 years
    d. less than 10 years
    e. over 10 years

16. Describe your personality.
    a. tense
    b. anxious
    c. cool, well-adjusted
    d. nervous
    e. excitable
    f. happy
    g. depressed

23. Leisure time activities before onset of pain [that is, husband's or wife's activities].
    a. sedentary (bridge, etc.)
    b. moderate activity (gardening, etc.)
    c. vigorous sports

25. Describe his or her [husband's or wife's] personality.
    a. tense
    b. anxious
    c. depressed
    d. cool, well-adjusted
    e. nervous
    f. excitable
    g. happy

26. Your relationship with spouse.
    a. excellent
    b. average
    c. poor

32. Your relationship with him [father].
    a. excellent
    b. average
    c. poor

37. Describe her [mother's] personality.
    a. tense
    b. anxious
    c. depressed
    d. cool, well-adjusted
    e. nervous
    f. excitable
    g. happy

44. Surgeries done to correct problem.
    a. laminectomy once
    b. laminectomy twice
    c. laminectomy three or more times
    d. laminectomy with fusion
    e. amputation
    f. freeing of scar
    g. removal of tumor
    h. other

46. When does pain occur?
    a. at rest
    b. sitting
    c. walking
    d. with working or lifting
    e. all the time
    f. less than 8 hours/day
    g. 8-16 hours/day
    h. during sexual intercourse

[Some of the words below describe your present pain. Select **ONLY** those words that best describe it. Use only a single word in each appropriate category—the one that applies best.]

62. a. flickering
    b. quivering
    c. pulsing
    d. throbbing
    e. beating
    f. pounding
    g. none of these

63. a. jumping
    b. flashing
    c. shooting
    d. none of these

64. a. pricking
     b. boring
     c. drilling
     d. stabbing
     e. lancinating
     f. none of these

65. a. sharp
     b. cutting
     c. lacerating
     d. none of these

68. a. hot
     b. burning
     c. scalding
     d. searing
     e. none of these

78. a. spreading
     b. radiating
     c. penetrating
     d. piercing
     e. none of these

85. [People agree that the following 5 words represent pain of increasing intensity. They are:
     a. mild
     b. discomforting
     c. distressing
     d. horrible
     e. excruciating]
     Which word describes your pain right now?

91. Your work history:
     a. same job over 5 years
     b. more than 2 jobs in past 5 years
     c. no work for 1 year
     d. no work for over 2 years
     e. retired because of age

Five times as many patients with "normal" personalities considered their spouses anxious as did the "severely disturbed" patients who were almost four times as likely to consider their spouses as "cool and well-adjusted"! Furthermore, 86 percent of "normal" patients considered their relationships with their spouses "excellent" and "average" while only 27 percent of the severely disturbed patients considered their marital bliss "average."

Interestingly too, four times as many "normal" patients have pain at rest as do "severely disturbed" patients, although among the adjectives used to describe pain we found only moderate differences between "severely disturbed" and "normal" individuals.

It is of considerable interest that only 38 percent of the

"severely disturbed" individuals had worked at the same job over five years, compared with 71 percent of the "normal" patients. Also 38 percent of the "severely disturbed" patients had done no work in over two years compared with 14 percent of the "normal" individuals, which seems to imply a greater tendency for better adjusted individuals to try to be employed. However, these statistics, which were obtained from the forms filled out by the patients, are highly suspicious since over 80 percent of our patients have had their pain for longer than two years and have not worked in that time.

Perhaps as interesting as those examination items which proved significant are those which seem to have *no* importance in determining personality alterations. Among others of little or no significance: the presence or absence of a lawsuit or claim; the frequency of sexual intercourse; the patient's relationships with his parents or his siblings; his relationships with his children; his type of work; his education; and prior psychiatric therapy.

The very same personality traits measured in test scores are, of course, also manifest in everyday behavior. As I've already pointed out, it is well-nigh impossible to decipher the cause-effect relationship between pain and concurrent personality changes. But what is apparent is that the pain patient's personality and his behavior are very much a part of his problem and consequently have to be reckoned with.

Finally, one really must have some technique for deciding how much pain the patient has. We will emphasize repeatedly that pain is a subjective problem and that there is no way of truly quantitating the amount of pain and that "pain threshold" is the same in most patients but tolerance is variable. The most useful technique which we have found is something we call the pain profile which was worked out by Dr. Jorge Picazza, Charles Ray, and myself:

PAIN SURVEY

Patient _____

Account No. _____

		Before Treatment	At Hospital Discharge	Follow up	Follow up	Follow up
	Date					
How much of the time is pain present?	0 = None					
	1 = 25% of time					
	2 = 50% of time					
	3 = 75% of time					
	4 = All the time					
How severe is your pain?	0 = None					
	1 = Mild					
	2 = Discomforting					
	3 = Distressing					
	4 = Horrible or excruciating					
Describe your physical activity in relation to what is physically possible.	0 = Normal					
	1 = Slightly Restricted					
	2 = Moderately Restricted					
	3 = Severely Restricted					
	4 = Totally Incapacitated					

44

Check your drug usage:

Up to 4 times/24 hrs.

	Date	Before Treatment	At Hospital Discharge	Follow up	Follow up
0 = None					
1 = Aspirin					
Salicylamide					
Ascriptin					
Bufferin					
Tylenol					
Acetaminophen					
Phenacetin					
APC's					
Pyrazolones					
2 = Barbiturates					
Chloralhydrate					
Meprobamate					
Valium					
Librium					
Placidy					
Paraldehyde					
Elavil					
Equagesic					

	Date	Before Treatment	At Hospital Discharge	Follow up	Follow up
Over 4 doses/24 hrs.	3 = Barbiturates				
	Chloralhydrate				
	Meprobamate				
	Valium				
	Librium				
	Placidyl				
	Paraldehyde				
	Elavil				
	Equagesic				
Up to 4 doses/24 hrs.	Darvon				
	Fiorinal				
	Codeine				
	Doriden				
	Zactirin				
	Percodan				
	Talwin tablets				
	Beer (up to 4 bottles or cans)				
	Whiskey of any kind (4 oz.)				

		Before Treatment	At Hospital Discharge	Follow up	Follow up
	Date				
Over 4 doses/24 hrs.	4 = Darvon				
	Fiorinal				
	Codeine				
	Doriden				
	Zactirin				
	Percodan				
	Talwin tablets				
	Beer (up to 4 bottles or cans)				
	Whiskey of any kind (4 oz.)				
	Morphine				
	Pantopon				
	Dilaudid				
	Demerol				
Any amount daily	Leritine				
	Methadone				
	Injectable Talwin				
	Over 4 beers/day				
	Over 4 oz. whiskey/day				

47

	Before Treatment	At Hospital Discharge	Follow up	Follow up	Follow up
Date					

Describe the effects of the pain upon your personality

0 = Normal, no effect, alert, cheerful, get along well.

1 = Slightly upset, irritable, disagreeable, moody, complaining.

2 = Moderately upset, unhappy, anxious, dull, uncooperative.

3 = Severely upset, quite depressed, bitter, desperate, withdrawn.

4 = Totally incapacitated, panicked, severely withdrawn, avoid everybody.

Using this questionnaire the usual patient entering our center gives himself a profile of 43342 on the five categories. The grade of 2 in the last category emphasizes the patient's tendency to minimize the effects of pain upon his personality. Actually, a grade of 3 would be more accurate in most patients. Interestingly, if patients are asked to grade their pain on the basis of 0 to 100—100 being the level of intolerable pain which would lead to suicide—the most commonly chosen number is 80. Using the pain profile, we see the usual patient awards himself sixteen possible points out of a possible twenty, that is 80 percent. These techniques at this moment offer the most useful criteria we've seen for evaluating the success of therapy. Ideally, total success or 00000 is sought, but since only 20 to 25 percent of our patients achieve this by the time they are discharged, it is essential that we have a range of values. Arbitrarily, therefore, we have ranked the profiles in this way:

Excellent: patients with a maximum of six total points on the pain profile. They may not have pain any more than 25 percent of the time; it may never be more than discomforting. The average excellent results has less than six points total.

Good: patients with a maximum of eight points, averages less than eight points; maximum is 22211.

Fair: patients with a maximum of ten points; maximum 22222 All other post-therapy scores are listed as failures.

Eighty percent of the patients treated at our center have initially been successes using these criteria. Obviously, however, the majority of the patients have not been "cured" or returned to full productive work. Indeed, our primary goal, when a patient has been an invalid for more than two years, is to break the drug-hospitalization-surgery cycle. Total rehabilitation is a much more complex problem and may require from one to three years for the most difficult patients. Some patients come to regard their suffering as a test of character, such as the woman who kept telling everyone who would listen, "I suffer in silence," or the man who kept repeating, "I have never lost my sense of humor"—although he had very little to laugh about and was, in fact, quite joyless. That these patients are getting an emotional pat on the back for being in pain is going to make management of their problems that much more difficult, if not impossible.

How ludicrous this game can become is seen in the case of a 38-year-old Caucasian man whose first of three back operations began six months after his wife presented him with a black child. Instead of resolving the very serious marital conflict, the patient became extremely depressed and at the very first minor injury developed into a chronic back invalid. It seems most unlikely that recovery can really occur until he comes to grips with the devastatingly inadequate marriage situation.

Of course, the complaint against a family member may be only one symptom of a pervasive personal discontent. But, in any case, relief from pain is going to require giving up, among others, the game of manipulating and blaming family members for problems.

The point of operant conditioning or behavior modification is to cut short the patient's pain game. The theory of this approach goes back to the Skinner box, which stirred up much debate and discussion. Actually, our approach is not quite so controversial; changing learned or practiced behavior plays an important part in many therapies and it need not be adversive or punishing.

The very fact that our patients seek help indicates that they are aware on some level that the pain game is unacceptable. While *we* cannot hope to restructure lives, pain management does require that the *patient himself* comes to terms with how much of his problem is operant or learned behavior.

Once that has been established, the patient needs to substitute new patterns of behavior. Instead of his usual behavior he is to substitute the behavior of a well person. This, of course, is accomplished by practice; even the patient's most sincere resolve to change his ways is usually not sufficient. Ideally, the patient's family, his employer, indeed his whole circle of acquaintances, should participate in learning new ways of responding to him, ways wnich reinforce well behavior and discourage pain patterns. The unfeasibility of this is obvious; we do, however, urge the spouses of our patients to take part in both the operant conditioning and the autogenics programs. Although marriage counseling is essential, financial considerations and riled emotions may make that impossible too. Speaking idealistically again, controlling pain and reestablishing marriages would be facilitated if both the patient and the spouse could spend at least two months in a carefully controlled program in which they could redefine their actions, reactions and their entire life scripts!

Our program of behavior modification is patterned after that of Dr. Wilbert Fordyce of the University of Washington. An essential ingredient of this kind of behavioral modification is the insistence that the patient cease complaining about pain. Since many pain patients are quite willing and able to discuss all their symptoms to everyone in sight, in order to discourage this concentration on suffering, my staff and the other patients are urged to ignore pain behavior and comments about pain and simply walk away if they continue. Only during consultations are patients permitted to speak to me about their pains and then they are limited to a brief statement of whether they are better, worse, or the same.

Perhaps the Pain Center situation gives patients some inkling of how they themselves appear. Certainly, those who are accustomed to taking center stage in any discussion of pain find it frustrating—and revealing, too—to find themselves in the company of several others who want to do the same thing. And they get some idea also of what pain behavior really looks like. One woman who played a perfect game of manipulation on all the other patients, requesting sweetly but pathetically that they fetch her water or adjust her pillows and so on (things they could hardly out of courtesy refuse to do) taught them a firsthand lesson in how the manipulative pain patient often relates to others.

At the very beginning of their stay at the rehabilitation center, patients are told that pain is not an emergency, and that we have no intention of treating it as such. They are also warned that suicide threats—even discussions or jokes about taking one's own life—are forbidden. Since threatening suicide has become for some patients the trump card of the pain game, the emotional blackmail that brings dramatic results in terms of sympathetic attention, we take a no-nonsense, harsh approach to it. Any patient who suggests that he is thinking about taking his own life is put immediately into the psychiatric ward and is sent directly home after his release from there.

Because he probably has been encouraged so often to take things easy, the pain patient very often has come to believe that his physical activity needs to be limited. Actually, if he has a strong desire to resume a normal life, then there really are no such limits (except for very heavy or strenuous labor); it is, in fact, totally conceivable that all pain patients can carry on a full and satisfying life without necessarily controlling the pain at all. When our center was part of the hospital, one of the cardinal rules was that patients had to come to the dining room for meals: being bed-ridden was not allowed. We have always had as part of our program certain exercise requirements intended to break down the patient's assumption that he cannot be active and at the same time to rebuild his physical condition which is most likely weakened by inactivity. When our patients were hospitalized, each was assigned to walk a certain number of hall laps (about one-half a city block) according to what the staff determined was physically possible for the particular patient's condition, and each day he was required to add one more lap to his regimen.

Since our program is limited to outpatient care, patients are encouraged to walk as much as possible. Some find, to their delight, that they can be much more active than they had realized and hence encouragement from us isn't even necessary. One patient recently hobbled into the clinic with a cane, claiming that he could hardly take five steps without it. On the third day in our program, he walked five *blocks* and back from a restaurant —without his cane!

Stationary bicycle riding is also assigned for two- to fifteen-minute periods, four times a day, with patients adding one minute per day. Supervised calisthenics are given twice a day (see Appendix) with patients increasing their participation as they increase their physical strength. We have also tried a "Swimnastics" or water exercise at the local YM-YWCA which has been most effective. Reminded that perseverence is essential, patients are urged to continue these exercises when they leave and to continue being physically active at home in order to rebuild, gradually over a period of months, the physical endurance of which everyone is capable. In order to dispel the notion that pain is a physical handicap, we encourage them to partake in all normal physical activities—except golf, horseback riding, bowling and heavy lifting, which should be added only when the body is in better condition. Upon returning home, many set up their own exercise programs preferably adding tried and tested programs such as Colonel Kenneth Cooper's Aerobics.

Taking drugs is also part of the pain patient's learned behavior and perhaps the most insidious of all his conditioned habits. Drugs almost invariably alter the patient's personality and decrease his physical activity. Yet, they do not satisfactorily relieve his pain; instead, tolerance (or tachyphylaxis) occurs within a few weeks which makes higher and higher doses necessary, increasing adverse effects with little additional benefit. Consequently, the patient can often add drug addiction to his list of problems.

Our particular philosophy regarding drugs is explained to the patients at the outset of their treatment, and it is made clear to them that gradual drug withdrawal is part of that treatment. Our premises are these: First, there are few drugs available which offer significant, lasting relief to the person with chronic pain. Scientific evidence will support this. Narcotics are to be avoided at all costs, and drugs of doubtful analgesic value are not used at all, no matter how commonly prescribed. Second, if drugs are used, combination products, which very often cause adverse side effects and are irrational mixtures anyway, are no better than single drugs; aspirin and acetaminophen are as effective as oral pentazoine, propoxyphene, etc., which are vastly overrated (full-color, medical journal ads not withstanding).

In order to help patients break the drug habit, we employ several methods. First, all medication is packaged in capsules of the same size, shape, and color; consequently, it is not difficult to change the drug dosage or even to switch the drug from one considered dangerous to another, safer one without the patient's knowledge. All tranquilizers (including those which can and do lead to physical and severe personality changes) and sedative-type drugs are converted to sodium amytal in dosages equivalent to the wide variety of mind-poisoners so commonly used. Antidepressants are converted to Elavil® which is taken at bed-time. Narcotics, which should be considered addicting, are converted to comparable dosages of methadone. Methadone was chosen because it can be taken orally and because it is a relatively long-acting, strong analgesic; it also provides a much milder degree of sedation and relatively few psychoactive effects. The synthetic analgesics (which produce such undesirable mental effects that it would have been better if they had gone undiscovered) and the patent medicine pain-killers are converted to aspirin or Tylenol® which the patients tolerate better and which are at least as effective in relieving pain anyway. The dosage of these drugs is gradually reduced: sodium amytal is withdrawn over a one- to two-week period; methadone is similarly slowly withdrawn in two and one-half weeks.

To further break up the drug habit, all medications, regardless of what they are, are given on a time schedule established by the doctor and they are not given whenever the patient thinks he needs them. There are several reasons for this, one of which is the hope that scheduled administration will disassociate in the patient's mind analgesia and other drug effects from pill-taking. Since the capsules look identical, the reduced dosage is not apparent to the patient. When the patient's drug dosage has been reduced to nothing and he has actually been taking a placebo for several days, he is made aware of that fact, and almost invariably patients will admit that their pain is no worse! More than likely they are feeling better because of the effects of increased physical activity, transcutaneous nerve stimulation, and other therapeutic techniques.

A schedule for the administration of drugs is also intended to curb the frequently irrational, often bizarre use of analgesics and tranquilizers. A few examples of actual cases should bear out the opinion that patients are not the best judges of how much medication they should be taking and how often. Several patients who had confirmed peptic ulcers were found to be taking large quantities of drug compounds containing aspirin, although they were aware that they should avoid aspirin and compounds containing aspirin. Similarly, three patients taking anti-coagulants were also taking high doses of aspirin and barbituates. Prior to admission to the center, one man was taking 50 mg. meperidine HCl tablets every two hours, supplemented with frequent meperidine injections and a half-dozen cans of beer per day. One woman was taking 45 to 60 tablets of a drug daily. The record was 60 mg. morphine injected every two and one-half hours! (A usual dose is 10-15 mg.)

No patients have demonstrated significant unpleasant reactions to our drug reduction program. Actually, our results can be put more positively than that. To use the two cases just mentioned as illustrations: The man was gradually withdrawn from meperidine and said he had *decreased* pain, although at that point we had done nothing more than withdraw him from drugs. After six weeks of behavior modification, he was discharged with an 80 percent reduction in pain. Eleven months later, he reported that he was completely pain free and had just received an award given to the employee with the greatest improvement in work attendance. In spite of the incredible doses, 45-60 tablets a day, the woman was converted to oral methadone (15 mg. every four hours) and gradually withdrawn without any difficulty whatsoever.

We never *recommend* that our patients take any drugs, but we have found three drugs which can be used—with certain limitations—in chronic pain cases: Elavil® (amitriptyline HC1), Dilantin® (diphenylhydantoxin) and Cobroxin® (cobra venom extract). In addition to being a substitute to antidepressants, Elavil® is used for obviously depressed patients and those who suffer from sensory deprivation pain, i.e. hypersensitivity in areas of partial nerve damage. Overall, about 25 percent of the patients—elderly ones, in particular—do not tolerate it; agitation, sleeplessness, drowsiness, confusion, postural hypotension, urinary retention, pedal edema, rashes or petechiae are all indications for withdrawing it. Since there is the possibility of intolerance, Elavil® is started at a bedtime dosage of 25 to 50 mg. and built up over a week's time to a top dosage of 150 to 200 mg. The patient should be told that his mouth becomes dry when he is taking the drug. Prolixin® which has been recommended by some therapists has proven highly unsatisfactory in our experience; drowsiness, confusion (and little benefit to boot) make it a poor choice. And in fifty patients who tried it with Elavil®, it proved no more effective that Elavil® alone. Thorazine® and most other mood-altering drugs have, after brief undesirable experience, proven poor choices for long-term help with chronic benign pain. If it seems to have a very beneficial effect, Elavil® may be maintained and even continued for another six months or so without mental obtundation. In sensory deprivation pain, Dilantin® may also be added, but it is not as likely to be useful as is Elavil®. Nevertheless, Dilantin® is one of the barely acceptable drugs for this limited type of pain.

The only other drug which we occasionally use in treating pain is Cobroxin®. This injectable (deep intramuscularly) extract of cobra venom has an extremely low rate of success and it requires daily shots for thirty to forty-five days before it is possible to determine for certain that it will be of any benefit. Therefore, in order not to confuse things when we're trying to determine which modality is effective, we usually do not start Cobroxin® until later. The only undesirable effects are instances of diplopia (double vision) or hives, both of which clear rapidly when the shots are discontinued. There have been reports of a beneficial effect of Cobroxin® upon mood; even though this is hard to document, it does not *worsen* personality or induce mental clouding. Perhaps for the patient whose drug orientation requires use of some type of medication, this is one of the simplest and safest "placebo" types to offer. However, having seen it most effective even in advanced cancer patients, I hasten to add that it is not *only* a placebo.

Finally, we flood our patients with vitamins in supertherapeutic dosages since many of them are not in very good physical condition anyway. At discharge we recommend that they take Enterra® or Maxivite®, one a day; Vitamin E, 400 units daily; and natural Vitamin C, 1 gram a day. This is a safe and effective vitamin supplementation and when we consider the effects of smog, physical and emotional stress, and food processing, it seems worthwhile to continue such recommendations. We also encourage our patients to improve the nutritional intake of the foods they eat. We suggest that they avoid sugar, keeping the level preferably to 1 percent of their total caloric intake and that they substitute honey as a sweetener; avoid hydrogenated oils and fats and use butter, pork lard, or vegetable cooking oils (safflower or corn oil, preferably) instead, and that they keep the ratio of polyunsaturated fats to 1 and 1/2 parts to 1 part saturated fat; avoid food additives like BHA and BHT and all processed foods; and that they include at least 50 grams and if possible 70 to 100 grams of protein per day. We discourage their smoking and taking caffeine through coffee, tea, and cola drinks. Alcohol should be limited to two or less ounces of whiskey or its equivalent per day.

Throughout our operant conditioning program, we try to break into the cycle of "ailing" behavior, to which the patient may have become addicted. In order to do this, we need to convince him that he is not a sickly invalid in need of extra consideration and care, unable to exist without a plentiful supply of analgesic drugs and sympathetic concern, but that he is rather, capable of a reasonably normal life. We also emphasize to each of our patients that good health is really *his* responsibility and that it is in part achieved and maintained by proper nutrition, adequate physical exercise, the avoidance of harmful habits, and good body-mind attunement which can be attained through autogenic training.

CHAPTER VI

Headache

Headache is, in most reported instances, the most common symptom in the world; and yet, in my own practice, the problem represents a relatively small part of the chronic pain program. On the other hand, it is quite obvious that headaches fall primarily into three categories, and here, of course, we are talking about the chronic headaches in which no apparent, significant organic abnormality is found; brain tumors and all other such possible causes of headache have been ruled out.

Migraine is the obvious and classic headache syndrome and so much has been written about it that my primary comments will be directed at the treatment of migraine. Interestingly, even in migraine headaches, we find that a huge percentage of patients have extreme tenderness of the transverse process or facet area of the vertebrae (C2-3). Pressure on that area will almost invariably reproduce the patient's symptoms or pain in the area where the patient's headache occurs. If the patient can be treated at the very beginning of a headache with an acupuncture needle placed in that area which corresponds roughly with gallbladder point 20, then pain relief is usually afforded. Similarly, application of external electrical stimulator to that point bilaterally at the beginning of the headache usually will abort the onset of a migraine headache. If external electrical stimulation in that area is not useful, then the stimulator may be applied bitemporally, bifrontally, or, with some precaution, over the caratoid sinuses.

We do not use drugs in the management of migraine headaches! Since a vast majority of patients with migraine have severe tension and autonomic distress, they tend to have generalized autonomic disturbances manifested by cold hands. Although a normal individual will usually have hands with a temperature in the mid-80s or higher, migraine patients usually have them somewhere in the 70s and occasionally even in the 60s. When migraine patients are taught to raise the temperature of the fingertips on command within a few minutes time up to a normal level of at least 93 to 96° F. then the frequency of the migraines tends to diminish rather markedly and if the patients will continually reinforce the practice by raising the temperature at the very onset of a headache, migraine can be extremely effectively controlled in about 80 percent of all sufferers. And a goodly percentage of the rest can have their migraines controlled by acupuncture and external electrical stimulation. Drugs should be reserved only for those patients who do not respond to this very simple and effective treatment program.

The other two kinds of headaches that are relatively common are tension headache and osteoarthritic cervical spine disease with referral reflex headache. Tension headache is best controlled by teaching the patients how to relax. This can be done with autogenic training and EMG (electromyograph) biofeedback reinforcement. Patients who have cervical osteoarthritic pain with referred reflex headache are the most difficult group of all, but again a combination of acupuncture, external electrical stimulation, autogenic training and biofeedback can be most helpful in helping these patients gain control over their headaches. Since drugs never relieve these patients adequately I do not believe that there is a place for drugs in the management of most chronic headaches. One might also consider the use of ice pack applications to the base of the skull or the suboccipital area at the very beginning of a headache and if used repeatedly these very·simple, mechanical techniques will help patients increasingly control their headaches.

NOTE REGARDING CHAPTERS VII AND VIII

The Pain Game is a unique overview of the trials and treatments of that phenomenon, unseen but keenly felt, PAIN. Strange as it may seem to the lay reader, it is also a rare opportunity for those in the medical field to consider within the covers of one book the alternatives for treatment of pain symptoms. In the following chapters the language is technical at times as treatments are outlined in detail, though many pain patients will understand a good deal of the terminology. In fact, it is hoped the book will help the patient to understand what a physician plans to do in treating pain and to decide whether he needs another physician's opinion before committing himself to a procedure.

For the lay reader, the important points to remember about the following chapters are: (1) Surgery for chronic pain is not an emergency and should be carefully considered because it cannot be "undone;" (2) Conservative (potentially harmless) forms of treatment should be considered first, before accepting a radical approach; (3) Some conservative treatments such as exercise, electrical stimulation and acupuncture may be unpleasant initially, but their long-term effects are often beneficial. They deserve an honest chance from the patient, for the alternatives, drugs and surgery, are far riskier.

CHAPTER VII

The Saga of the Back

There was a crooked man
Who walked a crooked style
He saw an orthopedist
Who sinisterly smiled.

Ahah! I have the answer
Your problem is quite clear
I diagnose a bulging disc
We'll remove it, have no fear.

The surgery was ended
The doctor got his fee
And now the disc that was removed
Is causing pain around the knee.

So that crooked man who still had
Pain and strife
Became another victim of a
Well-intended knife.

Unfortunately, this poem, written by one of my patients, comes all too close to the distressing truth. Most of our patients suffer from benign (nonmalignant) low back pain, and far too many have been subjected to the risky testing and therapeutic procedures intended for diagnosing and treating disc herniation. The fact that many of these same patients end up at our clinic—and the offices of other physicians as well, I'm sure—indicates the futility of that approach to cervical or lumbar spine problems.

It is my feeling that for the majority of our patients suffering from noncancerous chronic spinal pain, facet denervation or facet rhizotomy (a technique for radiofrequency localization and coagulation of articular nerves supplying the spinal facets) should be considered if the conservative methods of treatment such as acupuncture and external electrical stimulation prove ineffective in controlling back, sciatic and/or arm pain.

The classic ruptured disc with impaired straight leg raising, muscle weakness, deep tendon reflex changes and/or sensory damage, low back pain, sciatica, and positive myelographic (special contrast x-ray) findings has been treated successfully for thirty years with partial hemilaminectomy, removal of the ruptured disc fragment, and nerve root decompression. After Mixter and Barr described the ruptured disc and the means of treating it, most neurosurgeons and orthopedists became convinced that all back and sciatic pain must be due either to a ruptured disc or to psychosomatic disorders; the result: excessive and unnecessary back surgery. Despite the widespread use of myelography (an x-ray in which a special dye is injected into the spinal canal) as a diagnostic aid, at least one-third of neurosurgeons operated purely on clinical grounds. But even myelography, the test for herniated disc, has a 30 percent chance of being "false positive." Furthermore, it seems likely that this dye, Pantopaque®, is a major inciting cause of the often devastating cases of arachnoiditis (severe scarring of the nerve roots) complicating disc surgeries. Only when a safer, simpler approach fails should patients be subjected to such risky diagnostic tests as the myelogram or the discogram (the contrast material is injected directly into the disc) or to such therapeutic procedures as laminectomy, which would be justly stamped with the warning, "For use only in cases of rupture."

Extensive clinical experience suggests that actual disc rupture is rare. First of all, a rupture would mean a break *through* the annulus fibrosus of the nucleus pulposus, a highly elastic and semifluid tissue. For this to occur, the posterior longitudinal ligament must be at least stretched if not torn. Of the 300 patients we shall summarize here, most are failures of earlier lumbar surgery and most of them had been previously diagnosed as having ruptured discs. A review of the original operative notes for 250 patients who had previously been operated on elsewhere, however, reveals definitive reports of disc herniation in *only six* of them; in twenty others the information supplied is insufficient to make a diagnosis. In 224 patients the operative notes clearly indicated that the original pathology consisted of a bulging, degenerated disc, not a ruptured disc at all! For obvious reasons, disc removal failed to produce pain relief for these patients. Interestingly, we also found only one ruptured disc in 45 patients who had had no previous surgery, but who otherwise complained of back and sciatic pain very similar to that of the patients who had failed to benefit from earlier hemilaminectomy, disc removal and/or fusion. Luckily, these 44 people were able to avoid unnecessary back surgery! From the evidence I have seen of misdiagnosed cases, it is apparent why statistics indicate that a minimum of 30 to 40 percent of all patients who undergo laminectomy for a disc, which is only presumed ruptured, fail to achieve pain relief; and it is obvious too why great care should be exercised in a decision for surgical intervention.

The case history of one of our patients—reproduced here as it appeared in his physician's referral letter—emphasizes the sad reality of unjustified back surgery:

> This thirty-two year old man was admitted with complaints of back and leg pain for elective spinal fusion. He has suffered from pain in the back and both legs since 1953, when he fell off or through a bridge while in the Army. Following this injury, he suffered from pain mainly in the back and, after several recurrences, he was offered disc surgery at [an army hospital] six months after injury. He

refused surgery at that time and since then has had a succession of episodes of sudden back and leg pain with intervening periods of complete relief. He was admitted to this hospital for the second time for this complaint in August 1965, and after a trial of conservative therapy, he was readmitted and a myelogram was performed on September 24, 1965. *On the basis of the finding of a disc protrusion defect in the myelogram at L4-5 on the right, he was subjected to a disc excision at L4-5 from both sides.* It was felt at this time that this *disc protrusion* could well explain all of his symptoms. He did well for a *short* period after surgery, but has been having considerable back pain. At the time of this admission his major complaint was pain in the back and sides and there were no significant neurological findings. [Italics mine]

On the day following admission, he was taken to the operating room and, under general anesthesia, a posterior and posterolateral spinal fusion was done from L4 to S2 using bone taken from both posterior superior iliac spines.

Needless to say, a bulge or protrusion is not necessarily a rupture. Six months later, the patient complained of pain more intense than his pre-fusion pain and he was subjected to a surgical cordotomy. The following week a second cordotomy left the patient paralyzed in both legs.

Another case: a forty-two-year-old man was referred to us with a history of back pain after a fall from a horse in 1962. Within one year after his accident, he had already had two lumbar laminectomies with fusion, and yet *no* ruptured disc was found! Continued pain in 1966 led to "extension" of the laminectomy and repeated fusion. Within seven years, *fourteen* spinal operations (an average of one every six months) were performed from C4 to the sacrum. The surgeon felt that each procedure "amazingly" gave the patient pain relief; nevertheless, in time the pain simply moved up to the next highest level of intensity.

Unfortunately, such amazement is exceedingly common: in the same week that we admitted this man we also admitted two other patients with fourteen spinal operations. Our files are bulging with case histories in which both patient and surgeon opted too readily for surgery; and quite commonly an operation has been advised after the pain has continued for only a month or two even though there is no clear-cut myelographic or neurologic abnormality. It is bad enough that most patients require a six-month recovery period after a laminectomy to return to anything near their normal activity, but worst of all such surgery often leads to chronic pain much more severe than the original complaint.

Herniated disc in the cervical area is even less common than in the lumbar region. However, I have been distressed to see more and more frequently patients who have had one to five cervical vertebrae fused *just for neck pain*. Such a procedure is no more warranted or safe than a lumbar fusion; based as it is on such flimsy criteria for surgery, it probably leads to many more failures than successes. Even when there is, in fact, a ruptured cervical disc, surgery is indicated only when there is neurologic damage, not simply when there is pain. Very commonly, a severe degenerative disease of spaces above and below fusions make fusion of the neck as unworthy a procedure as a fusion of the lumbar spine, which is warranted only in cases of true fracture or dislocation.

As I've indicated, the classic syndrome of disc herniation is pertinent to only a small proportion of all patients complaining of chronic low back pain and sciatica. In most of our patients, neck, back, sciatic and/or arm pain is the result of subluxation, that is the partial dislocation or "slipping" of the spinal facets, which is brought on by the degeneration or bulging of a disc or discs. No wonder, for most patients suffering from low back and sciatic pain, that the customary attempts to relieve chronic symptoms by hemilaminectomy and disc removal not only fail, but they may make matters worse. In fact, such measures are ineffective in cases:

1. of chronic low back pain with or without sciatica, little or no motor, reflex, or sensory changes (patients suffering from this type of pain often have a virtually normal myelogram or a minimal abnormality of questionable significance);

2. of lumbar spondylosis with long-standing degenerative disc disease;
3. of pure "discogenic" pain;
4. of disc surgery failures who have undergone previous laminectomies with or without fusion.

Obviously, examination of the patient is crucial, since back pain might arise from any number of sources, e.g. nerve roots and the branches thereof, muscles, the periosteum, ligaments, or the joints, mainly the facet and the sacroiliac joint; the physician must be able to determine the area or areas involved. Since all back and/or leg pain began as an acute process, it is important to make the differential diagnosis on the basis of the pain at its onset which would more clearly define the problem area. The history itself is usually not that important, for most patients develop back pain during minimal stress, like twisting, falling, lifting small objects, or doing things which they may have done with ease many times before.

If the pain is lumbar, physicians must observe the patient standing, sitting and walking; and look for scoliosis, paravertebral muscle spasms and the favoring of one leg. Patients usually vary greatly in their abilities to flex the back. Similarly, straight leg raising may be limited to 10 degrees or the patient may be capable of a 90-degree flexion. When there is crossed pain (left leg or back pain when the right leg is raised, for instance), there is a much greater possibility of genuine nerve root impingement by a ruptured disc fragment.

Tenderness over one or more spinal facets or over the sacroiliac joint is common and of little value in differential diagnosis. Sensory changes are also notoriously incapable of yielding definitive information since "numbness" is seen in any area of pain. Varied degrees of "reflex" hypalgesia and hypesthesia are seen in many patients with back and/or sciatic pain and should not be construed as evidence of nerve root damage.

Muscle strength should also be checked carefully. Often there is a mild relative weakness because the pain limits effort. Subjective weakness is common to this kind of pain since "holding" of the muscles leads to apparent weakness or to apparent reflex changes. Only when there is unequivocal muscle weakness (most often evident in extension of the great toe or in dorsiflexion of the foot) is nerve root damage a likely possibility. Deep tendon reflexes are dependent on the state of relaxation of the patient; so useful information is gained only when a reflex is totally absent, which also would raise the question of possible nerve root damage.

X-rays of the affected spinal area will assist in ruling out compression fracture and metastatic cancer. A complete blood count should be done for general medical purposes and a blood sugar is necessary to rule out early diabetic neuropathy. But, if there is no significant muscle weakness and no bladder or bowel dysfunction, then there is no need to subject the patient to the discomfort and the risk of contrast diagnostic tests, *unless* conservative treatment has been given an *adequate* chance and that approach has reached an impasse.

Assuming that all the tests are normal and there is no definitive evidence of neurologic damage, then conservative management of this kind of pain is in order. At its acute stage, we prescribe bed rest for a day or two until the muscle spasms subside. Muscle relaxants, sedatives and analgesics are indicated only in extreme cases and then only for a brief duration of one or two days. During this period, ice packs and external electrical stimulation may offer symptomatic relief. As soon as the patient is reasonably comfortable, ambulation should begin; and gentle flexion and extension exercises can be added as soon as possible. Acupuncture may be of considerable benefit early in the course of back pain; if tenderness is limited to the sacroiliac joint, vigorous needling of the joint may be the most satisfactory treatment. Rarely, it may be necessary to inject long-acting steroids into a very irritated joint. Finally, if pain relief is not achieved by the fifth day, Marcaine® block (1 cc. of 0.25 percent) injected under X-ray control over the tender facets may be effective. While cervical traction may help in neck pain, relief of back and neck pain is less likely in pelvic traction; consequently, if no benefits occur within one week, traction is unlikely to be beneficial at all.

Similarly, lumbosacral supports have limited value and should not be continued beyond one month unless there is a fracture or dislocation. In Europe, spinal manipulation is an accepted therapy and in properly selected patients it may be the deciding factor in recovery.

If the patient has experienced pain and has been inactive and out of work for six months, he becomes increasingly resistant to conservative therapy. For such patients, facet rhizotomy may be the answer to relieving pain. If nothing else, it is safe and harmless, which is no small point in its favor.

For the management of neck and arm pain, I recommend that the treatment begin as conservatively as possible, with ice packs, acupuncture or acumassage, and external electrical stimulation employed more or less concomitantly. Even though traction is usually useless for lumbar pain, it may be helpful in cases of cervical pain. However, unless it offers considerable relief, it should not be continued for more than two days. If it is used, I would suggest eight to ten pounds of weight with the patient in traction for one hour and then off for the next, alternating the hours thus between 8 A.M. and 10 P.M. A cervical collar may be more effective than traction, but even so it should not be used for longer than one month.

The possibility of using some other technique for destruction of the facet nerves must be considered. Dr. Donlin Long has used hypertonic saline and we have now had experience in six patients using 33 cc. of 5 percent saline injected *on* the center of the joint, with subsequent injection of Depo-Medrol. It is too early to be certain of this approach except to note that it is quicker but leaves the patients for a week or ten days with more pain than the radiofrequency procedure does. Recently, we have also used 4% phenol in glycerine with excellent early success.

I would hasten to add, however, that in spite of our successes with the technique, facet denervation alone will not suffice in chronically disabled patients who must be taught behavioral and physical techniques essential for their return to a more active, normal life. The ultimate place in our therapeutic armamentarium for facet denervation requires further time and experience, but present indications are that it is safe, simple, and often very satisfactory. Indeed, it appears likely that the majority of back and sciatic pain syndromes are the result of mechanical alterations in the small facet joints and not the ruptured disc as so often has been assumed. Considering that, one of the most important contributions of facet rhizotomy may be its calling attention to structures other than discs as the sources of back pain.

Finally, it is worthwhile to consider the sacroiliac joint as a source of back and sciatic pain. When facet rhizotomy fails or seems of no value from preliminary facet nerve blocks, injection of the sacroiliac joints is worth considering. Many patients have obtained striking pain relief (even of sciatica) by this therapy. If it succeeds, 5 cc. 0.25 percent marcaine plus 40 mg. Depo-Medrol, injected *into* the sacroiliac joint under fluoroscopic control may be of great benefit. Such injections repeated about once every four to six weeks over a six-month period may lead to rehabilitation.

In summary, the saga of the back is not a closed story. Much remains to be learned. However, it is now quite apparent that ruptured discs play a relatively minor role in back and sciatic pain.

Many of the "recurrent disc" problems which plague neurosurgeons and discourage patients are actually epidural adhesions, often of great tenacity and almost bond hard. Even when decompression relieves these resurgent pains, there is great fear of a subsequent recurrence of the concrete encasement of nerve roots. Furthermore, many referring physicians and a greater number of patients fear disc surgery because of the reported failure rate; some patients continue to suffer because they are unwilling to accept such odds. Similarly, the thick collagenous investment of operated peripheral nerves sometimes is responsible for late neuropathy. A simple method for prevention of adhesions should be of benefit to many thousands of patients.

In January 1966, during surgery on a patient with extensive epidural adhesions, we were impressed by the generous epidural fat around an adjacent unoperated nerve root. We, therefore, elected to transplant subcutaneous fat to the L5 nerve root which had been freed of adhesions. The patient, a 32-year-old telephone lineman, returned to work within six weeks, a feat he had been unable to do after his original disc surgery. He had no further recurrence.

Even the most emaciated patient has a covering of peridural fat around the spinal nerve roots. Presumably this fat is essential for mechanically smooth gliding of nerve roots while the spine is moving.

The frequency of epidural adhesions has been well documented. Only one paper has dealt with therapy for this problem significantly. Mayfield and O'Brien reported the use of artificial grafts in those patients with dural constriction from epidural scar. We are unable to find any previous report of a method for *prevention* of the syndrome.

One paper has reported the use of fat implants in reconstructing "deep depressing scar of the cheek and forehead." The authors reported excellent long-term cosmetic results; and in one of their cases microscopic examination revealed good preservation of the transplanted fat. Methods for prevention of scar in other areas of the body are not necessarily feasible or safe in epidural areas.

It is obviously too early to determine whether epidural fat implants will totally abolish the late epidural adhesions so commonly seen in the past. To date we have had no patients of the current series return with this problem. Undoubtedly pain will recur in patients with truly new ruptured discs, with unstable intervertebral or paravertebral joints, and with arachnoiditis. However, it is hoped that epidural fat implants will prevent one of the most exasperating causes of disc surgery failure, epidural adhesions.

Furthermore, fat is an excellent coating for nerve grafts and may prevent perineural scarring in other forms of peripheral nerve surgery. This may be of particular value when there is overlying tissue necrosis as transplanted fat in this situation can survive and act as a protective layer to underlying inert nerve grafts. Since epidural and peridural scars are often invoked as "causes" for continuing pain, we believe this simple, safe technique deserves widespread use.

If you do have to have a laminectomy, it seems worthwhile to discuss with your surgeon the desirability of such fat implants. I would not want a laminectomy without!

CHAPTER VIII

Mechanical Therapy

Electroanalgesia

Pain can be lessened or inhibited by non-painful stimulation applied either directly or remotely. Electrical stimulation or electrical analgesia (transcutaneous, percutaneous, and intra-spinal) is especially useful in headaches, acute sprains, causalgia (that is, the burning sensations caused by injury to peripheral nerves) and childbirth. Indeed, I feel that over 75 percent of deliveries could be performed relatively painlessly and safely under electroanesthesia.

Actually, the use of electricity for pain relief is not a new practice: The first recorded use of electroanalgesia is over 2000 years old. Although some knowledge of the electrical powers of certain fish was known to the ancient Egyptians and even to Hippocrates, the first use on record occurred in A.D. 46 when Scribonius Largus, a Roman physician, claimed to be able to cure the pain of headache and gout with the energy produced by electrical fish. Thus, this ancient physician and contemporary of Pliney, might be considered the father of the body of medicine devoted largely to electrical therapy. The electric fish were used intermittently for a variety of illnesses until about 1745 when the advent of the Leyden jars ushered in the beginning of neurophysiology. Most initial experiments centered around the use of electrical shock to elicit skeletal muscle contractions, and early attempts were made to control paralyzed limbs, which is still an area of interest today. The practical harnessing of electrical energy was not accomplished, however, until Franklin's isolation of frictional electricity; and shortly thereafter, the evolution of galvanic and faradic currents spawned the electrotechnology of today.

By the mid-1800s the fact that electricity could be of use in pain control was understood, but the rapidly growing drug industry and the somewhat slower-moving field of engineering design managed to eclipse scientific evidence. Nevertheless, as so often happens whenever an important truth is suppressed, there were people who did recognize the inherent benefits of electrotherapy and the result was the faddish promotion of electrical belts and gadgets of every conceivable design which were widely manufactured and sold through lay advertisements and by door-to-door salesmen purporting that these devices could cure almost every disease. Their promoters added to the appeal of their gadgets by incorporating metaphysical and occult philosophy into their instruction books, which are to a physician more fascinating and delightful reading than a 1908 Sears catalogue. Relying upon testimonials of satisfied users, the promoters emphasized the magic of electricity and claimed, completely illogically, of course, that it could cure pain, fatigue, emotional problems, and every illness from acne to cancer.

Not all these therapeutic devices were nonsense, however. There were at least two lasting contributions made during this period. One was the demonstration that atrophy of paralyzed muscles could be prevented by regular electrical stimulation. The other was the introduction of diathermy, the induction of heat by electricity, and its widespread use, initially, to destroy diseased tissue. In this was the genesis of electrocautery, an essential technique in modern neurosurgery, and of radio-frequency produced lesions. In addition, the era of internal stimulation began around 1900 with the demonstration that electrical current could affect bladder contractions. The clinical perfection of devices for this purpose has not yet been achieved, although some progress has been made.

In spite of these therapeutic contributions, in the 1940s the Food and Drug Administration (FDA)—a veritable bureaucratic dinosaur—exercising far more restraint than it ever has over the drug industry, put an end to this enterprise. Using such tactics as suggesting that internal electrodes designed to treat hemorrhoids were pornographic, they forced every American manufacturer of external battery-powered stimulators out of business, even though no harm in using these gadgets was ever reported. The only company allowed to continue in business was Electreat® but with certain restrictions: it was not allowed to advertise that its products can relieve pain, even though that claim has been empirically proved by over 300,000 users of the devices.

However, the development of electricity in cardiology has been remarkable, in spite of the establishment's customary disdain for and distrust of new concepts. As early as 1900 electrical shock was known to be capable of reversing ventricular fibrillation. Up until the last few years, cardiac physiology was far ahead of all other medical fields beginning with and largely as a result of the use of percutaneous cardiac pacing which was demonstrated in 1927. Since then technical advances have lead to entirely new designs every few years. Consequently, the cumbersome implantable pacemakers which were in their infancy over fifteen years ago have been updated by more refined and complex designs. Cardiac pacemaker electronics, a huge field in itself, has spurred on the development of the related fields of bioengineering and biomedical engineering and of the growth of the whole medical electronics industrial complex.

The neurosciences, on the other hand, were content with the development of simple electronic feedback machinery, e.g. the EMG (electromyograph), EEG (electroencephalograph) and occasional depth recordings, and psychiatrists were excited, temporarily, by electroshock therapy. In spite of Galvani's demonstration almost two hundred years ago that electrical nerve stimulation led to muscle contraction, and in spite of the tremendous advances in neurophysiological understanding of the nervous system which have occurred during the last thirty years, there was no practical modulation of the nervous system until Melzack and Wall's gate theory of pain caught the imagination of neurosurgeons in 1965. When I heard the theory, I postulated that pain might be controlled by the electrical stimulation of the dorsal columns of the spinal cord; and in 1967 we inserted the first human dorsal column stimulator (DCS).

The gate theory of pain (the details of which are still controversial) emphasizes the natural balance of neural activity between the large and small sensory fibers; the amount of sensory input transmitted to the brain at any one time is influenced by the ratio of activity of these peripheral nerve fibers. Observations, which have been mostly empiric, have demonstrated that the large beta fibers do not themselves carry pain information, whereas the C fibers do. Thus, physical pain results whenever there is increased C fiber input, mostly from nerve irritation, or whenever these fibers are selectively damaged in surgery, or in *herpes zoster,* etc. It is probably the disturbed balance which is responsible for the various pains of anesthesia dolorosum, post-cordotomy dysthesia, paraplegic pain, the thalamic syndrome and phantom limb pain.

The balance between the beta and the C fibers occurs at many synapses (gates) through the usual neuromodulation techniques of inhibitions and excitations. These gates may, however, be influenced. If the large fibers which conduct sensation but not pain are peripherally stimulated, the spinal cord mechanism is overloaded and the activity of the smaller, pain-conducting fibers is inhibited. The autonomic nervous system through many descending messages from the brain and spinal cord can also control the sensory input balance; but the preponderance of control comes from the limbic system, the central computer which is the seat of emotions and feelings.

Our clinical use of this knowledge has led to the application of electrical stimulation to almost all parts of the body. When pain is focal, we first try external electrical stimulation or transcutaneous nerve stimulation (TNS) of the affected region. If this does not succeed, and occasionally it only accentuates the pain, we stimulate areas surrounding the painful part or we stimulate through needles inserted into the area. If this also fails to afford pain relief, we resort to stimulation of numerous unrelated regions. Clinically, this becomes an elaborate project and it is not always successful; nevertheless, the procedure is so safe that it bears careful consideration before other, more hazardous therapy is attempted.

If it is not possible to control adequately the spinal cord's transmission of pain with external stimulation, the implantation of electrodes, under proper circumstances, might be considered. Occasionally, peripheral nerve stimulation (PNS), that is, implantation of stimulators around major nerve trunks with subcutaneous radio-receivers may offer relief; or, but only after careful consideration has been given to various indications and contraindications, the DCS, or dorsal column stimulation, might be considered. However, we feel that transcutaneous stimulation should be tried for at least two weeks before consideration is given to an implanted device. And indeed, I recommend six months of autogenic training before a final decision is made.

The transcutaneous nerve stimulator (TNS) was originally intended to be used as a trial stimulator preceding the DCS implantation. We believed it necessary that patients have some idea what kind of sensations to expect before the actual implant surgery was performed; for that reason, we resurrected the ancient Electreat®, which was patented in 1918 by a naturopath, as a screening device for patients being selected to undergo implantation of the DCS. The pain relief achieved from this simple, archaic device in its own right was so marked that in 1967 we urged the development of a miniature solid-state external transcutaneous stimulator. That development was delayed until 1971. Finally, pressure from neurosurgeons who had found the cumbersome Electreat® model at about the same level of sophistication and efficiency as the Wright Brothers' airplane, helped rush the development somewhat to what could be called the DC-3 level by 1974. But TNS models comparable to the jet engine 727 and 747 have still to be created. Nevertheless, the equipment currently available, cumbersome as it might be, is still capable of controlling most acute pain and a significant number of chronic pains.

The device itself is fairly simple: a pulse generator, a pair of electrical cables and a pair of electrodes which are attached with an adhesive to the patient's skin. So far what really has determined whether the device is successful or not is the persistence of the patient and the staff in adjusting and readjusting the site of the electrodes and the frequency of the pulses. This method of trial-and-error can be time-consuming. It is essential, however, that repeated trials of stimulation be done and the response should be reproducible on numerous occasions. Stimulation should be done at the patient's comfort level for thirty to one-hundred-twenty minutes at least four, and up to twelve times per day. Occasionally even a low rate (even one pulsation per second) stimulation is most satisfactory, but most patients choose 50 to 100 pulsations per second. Stimulation should be adjusted up to a strength which *causes* pain and then lowered slightly to the *comfort* level. Patients should then adjust the frequency of pulses to test various combinations. It is important to remember that the pulse frequency of greatest pleasure is not necessarily the same as that for most satisfactory analgesia.

Patients should try the electrodes on one stimulation site for at least twenty-four hours before rejecting it; if pain relief is not achieved in that period of time, the patient should move on to test another site. Generally, the entire area of pain should be tested first since that is the most likely to offer relief. In some extremely sensitive areas, however, electrodes are best placed on either side of the painful region. If application to the painful area itself offers no results, the surrounding area should be tried. Finally, if both focal stimulation and stimulation of concentric sites prove ineffective, we have our patients try the various points illustrated in the following figures. These sites include the major nerve trunks and the major acupuncture points as well, so there is an adequate chance to evaluate most possibilities for reflex inhibition of pain.

SUGGESTED SITES FOR ELECTRODE PLACEMENT

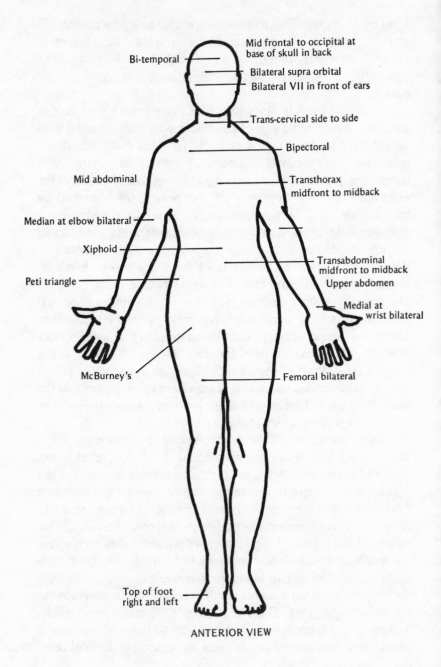

Bi-temporal

Mid frontal to occipital at base of skull in back

Bilateral supra orbital

Bilateral VII in front of ears

Trans-cervical side to side

Bipectoral

Mid abdominal

Transthorax midfront to midback

Median at elbow bilateral

Xiphoid

Transabdominal midfront to midback
Upper abdomen

Peti triangle

Medial at wrist bilateral

McBurney's

Femoral bilateral

Top of foot right and left

ANTERIOR VIEW

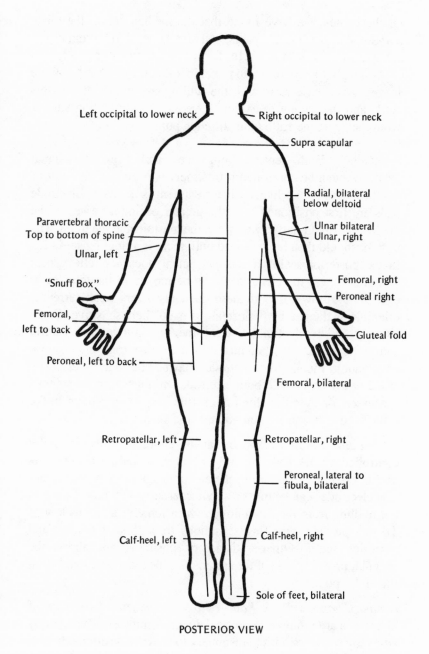

Left occipital to lower neck

Right occipital to lower neck

Supra scapular

Radial, bilateral below deltoid

Paravertebral thoracic Top to bottom of spine

Ulnar bilateral Ulnar, right

Ulnar, left

"Snuff Box"

Femoral, right

Peroneal right

Femoral, left to back

Gluteal fold

Peroneal, left to back

Femoral, bilateral

Retropatellar, left

Retropatellar, right

Peroneal, lateral to fibula, bilateral

Calf-heel, left

Calf-heel, right

Sole of feet, bilateral

POSTERIOR VIEW

Of these sites, we have found that the median nerve, the ulnar nerve, the upper cervical paraspinal and the top and bottom of the spine are the ones most useful for remote stimulation.

Although it is important to remember that the success or failure in any given case rests with the willingness of the doctor, his staff, and the patient to explore a variety of stimulation sites, I would suggest the following stimulus points:

Headache. Both tension, migraine, and even port-spinal headaches can be controlled if treatment is begun *at the onset* of pain; success is less likely when treatment is delayed. Electrode pads are first positioned over the greater occipital nerves in the nuchal line about halfway between the mastoid and the inion. The current should then be increased until there is a tingling sensation in the posterior scalp. If this placement does not relieve pain within minutes, the electrodes may be moved to the temples or over the eyebrows. In both these sites only a very weak current is tolerable as the nearby periosteum is exquisitely sensitive. Occasionally, bilateral stimulation of the region over the carotid sinuses is successful, but this should be first tried under close observation. Finally, the electrodes may be placed transcervically at C2 or lower; or with both electrodes midline over the spinous processes, or over the Hoku point (the acupuncture point in the right hand between the thumb and first finger).

Neck Pain. Most neck pain can be either partially or totally controlled by the TNS, but very often the deciding factor in its usefulness is whether or not the electrodes are too cumbersome. The electrodes can be moved about transcervically on the neck in the midline from the inion down. Occasionally, a site as low as T6 can produce vibrating sensations throughout the neck and posterior scalp. Other satisfactory positions are above the scapula, on either side of the spine, over the brachial plexus, or at the Hoku point.

Lumbar/Thoracic Back Pain. In some patients two pairs of electrodes are required to cover the pain completely. We start by adjusting the electrodes paraspinally to find the position which is comfortable and effective for the patient. Usually, this placement proves satisfactory, but if not, midline placement should be tried. If that too proves ineffective, we try the top and bottom of the spine, the ulnar nerves, the median nerves, the sciatic nerves, and the peroneal nerves. Occasionally, the pain is strongest at the sacroiliac junction, or in a thin individual, stimulation of the tender area itself is painful; in that case, the electrodes must be placed slighly lateral or cephalad to the trigger point. Incidentally, one female patient with chronic use of lateral chest stimulation recently reported marked breast enlargement.

Sciatica. For sciatic pain, extensive testing of a variety of positions to find the best combination for the individual patient is often necessary. Often, however, the most successful positioning is the placement of one electrode pad just to one side of the lower lumbar spine at about L5-S1 and the other over the sciatic nerve at the gluteal fold, or beside the head of fibula over the peroneal nerve, or on the sole or top of the foot, or over the femoral nerve. Alternatively, the transcervical sites or the ulnar or median nerves may be successful. Occasionally, adequate sciatic tingling can be accomplished only by stimulating through a probing needle (22 gauge or smaller) inserted into either the buttocks or the mid-posterior thigh near the peroneal nerve, or paraspinally at L4-5 or L5-S1.

Arm, Hand or Finger Pain (Including Causalgia). Adequate stimulation for these kinds of pain can most often be achieved with one electrode over the anterior forearm and the other either on the palm, on the dorsum of the hand, over the ulnar nerve at the elbow, in the axilla or over the brachial plexus above the clavicle. Careful placement of electrodes centered over the median and the ulnar nerves will usually give not only pain relief, but even anesthesia of the hand. In some individuals, it is necessary that one of the exploring electrodes (or sometimes, through rarely, both) be a small needle inserted near the median or ulnar nerves at the elbow or the wrist; even more rarely, it may be necessary to insert the needle near the supraclavicular brachial plexus. Sometimes, areas throughout the neck might also be found effective. We have not yet tried the ears as major stimulation sites despite the tremendous enthusiasm of some of our Chinese colleagues for "aurioculotherapy."

Rectal, Vaginal and Perineal Pain. Only occasionally can surface electrodes, one placed over the perineum itself and the other over the sacrum, provide adequate pain relief in these cases. In some patients a bipolar electrode needs to be inserted directly into the rectum or vagina to deliver stimulation to the appropriate area. Almost invariably, adequate stimulation can be achieved by stimulating a needle inserted directly anterior to the coccyx with the indifferent electrode placed either in the hand or over the sacrum.

Arthritis. For arthritic pain, the placement of electrodes on either side of the affected joints is most effective, especially so at the knees, hips, shoulders and spine. Occasionally, more diffuse stimulation, such as the stimulation of the major nerve trunks supplying the area, may be necessary.

Bursitis. For bursitis, the electrodes should be placed on either side of the most tender area, not directly over it.

Face and Dental Pain. Electrodes are adjusted over the area of pain, either supraorbital, infraorbital, mental, greater occipital or in combinations of these. In about one-third of the patients, needle stimulation is considerably more effective than surface stimulation. Occasionally, needles are inserted paraspinally at C1-2 out near the transverse processes. In some dental pain it is preferable to place electrodes directly on the gums to achieve adequate analgesia.

Abdominal Pain. One electrode may be placed over the epigastrium while the other is positioned over or near the thoracic spine. For example, with gallbladder pain, one electrode is placed in the right upper quadrant and the other over the area of referral pain in the right posterior shoulder area.

Labor. Two electrodes can be adjusted over the sacrum or the paralumbar area which most satisfactorily controls the low back pain of childbirth. Additional exploring electrodes can be placed over the nasion or the bilateral anterior forearms, paraspinally at C1-2, over the inion, or in a variety of sites over the abdomen or the lower thoracic spine. For the terminal stages of labor, considerable trial may be necessary to find the best site for electrode placement; at the stage of perineal pain, coccygeal needles or flexible electrodes have been found to be most satisfactory.

Potentia. Electrical stimulation may be quite beneficial for cases of impotentia. The electrodes should be placed just posterior to the scrotum and over the anterior base of the penis. Occasionally, the electrodes may be placed on either side of the base of the penis; or, in rare cases, one electrode may be inserted into the rectum. When stimulation alone proves inadequate, ice packs may be applied to the penis for between five and fifteen minutes during the stimulation. These techniques are extremely effective in high cord level paraplegics and may be of great benefit in some psychogenic impotentia.

Tension and "Nerves." With electrodes held in the palms of both hands, strong, but not painful, stimulation can be used for ten to fifteen minutes from four to ten times per day. Many anxious patients find this method of relieving tension as effective as tranquilizers; it is even more effective if the patient also jogs five to ten minutes four times a day (with gradual build-up to tolerance).

Post-operative Pain, Acute Wounds, Lacerations, Sprains, etc. Electrodes may be placed from one to two inches on either side of the wound or above and below it. Occasionally it is preferable to stimulate the major nerve supply to the painful area or to insert needles on either side of the painful spot. Post-operative electrical stimulation also appears to reduce the incidence of complications following abdominal procedures, to stimulate gastrointestinal tract function following surgery, and to reduce the amount of time spent by the patient in intensive care. Atelectasis is almost entirely eliminated and the incidence of ileus is markedly reduced.

Neurologic Deficit. In stroke patients and in individuals with leg or arm weakness, electrodes may be applied either on the palm of the hand or on the sole of the foot; on the palm and the shoulder; on the sole and the peroneal nerve. We have used stimulation at the maximum comfort level for two to ten hours per day in ten patients in order to increase awareness of paralyzed limbs. Subjectively, we think muscle power and spasticity are improved by such stimulation.

Angina Pectoris. Transcutaneous stimulation has given pain relief in cases of angina pectoris and after myocardial infarction. Most importantly, however, such therapy should be carried out *only* in hospitals and preferably in intensive care units. Such stimulation has been used in patients with cardiac pacemakers, but certain demand pacemakers may be affected adversely, so manufacturers advise against such use in pacemaker patients. Primarily the TNS must never be used *near* the pacemaker.

Post-herpetic Pain. One of the most satisfactorily treated pains, post-herpetic pain may cease after three to six months of pain control. Electrodes may be positioned on either side of the scar. Occasionally, two sets of electrodes may be needed and it may be necessary to explore paraspinally in the area leading to the painful site.

The effectiveness of the TNS has depended most of all upon the persistence in its application. About 2,000 of our patients have used the device and we have not seen any significant complications. In 5 to 10 percent of the patients, there was minor skin reaction either to the adhesives used to hold the electrodes in position or, rarely, to the electrodes and/or their coupling ionic chemicals. Two patients who placed the electrodes in precisely the same spot for six months developed neovascularization which promptly subsided when they began slight variations in positioning. In one study, we treated 136 patients who were suffering with various kinds of chronic pain with external stimulation. Of these patients 102 received moderate benefits and 30 required no other therapy beyond external electrical stimulation. In a more extended study of 750 patients we achieved the following results, which I think should serve as encouragement for further development of this kind of pain control:

PERCENTAGE OF PATIENTS ACHIEVING PAIN RELIEF

	Poor	Fair or Incomplete	Good to Excellent
Acute (surgical wounds, fractures, sprains, etc.)	20	20	60
Parturition			
Back Pain	25		75
Perineal Pain	80	10	10
CHRONIC PAIN			
Post herpetic	25	15	60
Phantom limb	40	35	25
Back Pain } Representing 60% of chronic patients	25	50	25
Sciatic Pain }	60	30	10
Neck Pain	50	25	25
Headaches	60	20	20
Arm & Hand Pain (including causalgia)	25	25	50
Diffuse Pain	80	10	10
Face Pain	50	25	25

Peripheral nerve stimulation (PNS) may prove beneficial whenever surface stimulation fails to provide relief from pain, but does not provide a disagreeable sensation. For pre-implant testing, we usually use the two parts of a disposable #20 gauge spinal needle as the two electrodes and insert them *just to touch* the nerve and to evoke referred tingling throughout the distribution of the nerve. Stimulation, which is under the patient's control, is then continued for thirty to sixty minutes. If pain relief is excellent this procedure is carried out in at least two subsequent trials. If we are in doubt as to its effectiveness, we insert flexible electrodes (the percutaneous DCS electrodes suffice for this purpose) near the nerve and allow the patient to test this kind of stimulation for one to four days. Only when 95 to 100 percent of the pain is repeatedly relieved do we recommend the implantation of a peripheral nerve stimulator (PNS). To date, we have had rather limited experience, with 22 implantations, 16 of which were on the sciatic nerve. Despite the pre-implant test results, only 12 of these 22 patients have achieved satisfactory pain control.

One of the most successful cases of PNS implant was also one of the most complicated and, initially, disappointing. A 45-year-old woman presented with a five-year history of back and left sciatic pain which was greatly aggravated by three surgical procedures. In 1973, a left sciatic nerve stimulator was implanted after extensive preoperative testing. Although the electrode was placed just below the sciatic notch the patient felt stimulation only from the popliteal area down. As has been our custom, the radio-receiver was placed in the lateral thigh. Although the pain was partially relieved, an intense sympatomatic irritation developed at the receiver site. Even after six months the skin over the receiver was slightly erythematous, swollen, and exquisitely hyperesthetic. Aspiration of the area revealed no fluid except one drop of tissue juice which was sterile. Finally, in desperation, we removed the receiver, coated it with bone-wax in order to reduce possible "allergic" reaction and replaced it in the left lower quadrant of the abdomen. Immediately after surgery, the patient felt the stimulus *up to the gluteal fold* which afforded her almost total pain relief. The new receiver site has since been free of pain and the hypersensitivity of the original receiver site cleared slowly with considerable mechanical stimulation (slapping and ice rubs). The patient has since been able to return to work. The success in this case raises the question of whether improvement might be possible in the other PNS patients as well by repositioning the electrodes and/or the receiver.

The concept of the DCS or dorsal column stimulation originated in 1965 after I read Melzack's and Wall's gate theory of pain. After laboratory confirmation of the concept, clinical use of the device began in 1967: in April of that year, I implanted the first human DCS. By 1971 neurosurgeons were more optimistic about its success than experience had suggested was reasonable; and by 1973 at least three companies were manufacturing a variety of DCS electrodes, none of which had been proven effective by the five-year standard I would consider essential for any sort of confidence or assurance.

Theoretically speaking, the dorsal columns offer the ideal stimulus site since they represent the only anatomical separation of beta fibers from other sensory fibers; therefore, electrical stimulation at that level offers an excellent opportunity for pain control. From a practical standpoint, however, there are inherent risks in the major surgical procedure of implantation. The complications we encountered have been, by and large, mechanical. There are, however, other major handicaps. For one, prior cingulumotomy or cordotomy make dorsal column electro-analgesia difficult if not impossible. In addition, there is also the possibility of misjudging a patient's suitability for this method of pain control.

The physiologic basis for the DCS has not as yet been proven by clinical studies; nevertheless, considerable further work by Willis, Sances *et al.*, and Richards *et al.* has confirmed the principle and suggests some physiologic mechanisms. The mechanical requirements for a perfect DCS system are both difficult to define and difficult to meet. Many of the complications of the DCS, as I've said, have been mechanical in nature. Major problems in electrode design have led to failure of the system in half of our patients; serious, potentially avoidable, and, fortunately, reversible complications occurred in 5 percent.

In no other neurosurgical procedure is careful selection of candidates so crucial. For that reason, I have recommended that the following conditions be met:

1. The patient have no serious emotional problems. We administer the MMPI (Minnesota Multiphasic Personality Inventory) to all our patients. We use this test to determine, in part, which patients have emotional difficulties and to what extent. People with chronic pain commonly have elevated scores on the hysteria, depression, and hypochondriasis scales, so we do not consider a slight elevation as indicative of serious emotional

disturbance. If the elevation is above 70 (that is, two standard deviations above the mean), however, we would undertake the DCS implant only with the greatest caution. Also, an elevation of any other scale other than these three is taken as forewarning of probable failure. At one time, we also took into account the opinion of a psychiatrist, who had experience with chronic pain patients, in determining the probability of successful pain relief in individual cases. However, the psychiatrist's opinion in itself was insufficient; interestingly, we found the surgeon's judgment on the patient and the patient's motivation even more reliable in determining probable success. In my own case, I would not implant a patient until I personally felt that he had a good chance of responding to treatment, no matter what the other criteria suggested.

2. The patient who has had cingulumotomy not be considered at all, and that the one who has been cordotomized be screened with even greater caution than usual. Patients who have had cord damage or who have had extensive posterior root sections should be considered only if percutaneous DCS affords excellent pain relief for at least twenty-four hours, and preferably longer.

3. The trial of transcutaneous electrical stimulation be carried out for at least one month and that it prove, first of all, the sensation is acceptable to the patient. Five percent of patients dislike the electrical sensation and find it more unpleasant than their pain; obviously they should not be implanted, most of them are hysterical. In other patients, partial or total pain relief can be accomplished with external stimulation, and in those cases DCS is not even necessary. Only through this testing period can the patient's acceptance of a "gadget" be determined. Finally, and importantly, the trial period also allows the patient and the physician to determine the degree of pain relief possible through electrical stimulation.

Percutaneous dorsal column stimulation should be done as a final test or whenever adequate stimulation of the painful region cannot be accomplished externally; it can be accomplished either by the direct needle technique of Adams and Hosobuchi, or preferably by a floating flexible electrode which can be adjusted and used for several days. Such stimulation is essential for deciding the possibility of success in paraplegics and patients with thalamic pain syndrome or whenever there is any question concerning the patient's relief from transcutaneous stimulation.

4. All patients have a trial period of operant conditioning during which they also test various mechanical methods of pain control. If that fails, they should have a minimum of six months of autogenic training and biofeedback. If they are not motivated enough to try these methods of self-control, they are probably not emotionally equipped for the DCS. Furthermore, if the basic personality and environmental abnormalities which prevailed when the patient became an invalid are not modified, long-term pain relief is not likely. Cancer patients should be the only ones excepted from this preliminary test period, although they too should be encouraged to partake in self-control programs.

A definition of success and failure is always controversial, particularly in something as subjective as feelings of pain and pain relief; but for purposes of determining the success of the DCS we used the Pain Profile described earlier. In this survey, the patient defines the extent of his pain according to five different criteria: the amount of time the pain is present, the severity of the pain, the physical activity of which he is capable, the effects of pain upon his personality, and his drug usage. He grades his pain in each of these areas from 0 to 4—the 0 indicating no discomfort and a total score of 20 (that is, a grade of 4 in each category) indicating the maximum level of pain and disability.

In a group of 80 patients who received the DCS, the total pre-implant score on the average was 17 and all the patients graded both the amount of time they experienced pain and the degree of their pain as 4, the maximum level. In order to judge how much relief they received from the DCS we classified, arbitrarily, those as "excellent" who had, after the implant, a total score of 6 or less—with pain no more than 25 percent of the time (a score of 1) and the degree of pain no more than discomfort

(2), that is a maximum of 3 points on those two scales. We considered those patients as "fair" or partial successes if their total score was no more than 10 points, and if they had discomforting pain (2) no more than 50 percent of the time (2), or else they had distressing pain (3) less than 25 percent of the time (1), that is they had a maximum of 4 points on those two scales.

Using these criteria for judgment, the DCS yielded the following later results for our group of eighty patients:

Excellent pain relief	12
Fair pain relief	25
Failures (14 of these late)	43

In contrast to these figures are the initial results which were determined within six months after the implantation:

Excellent pain relief	20
Fair pain relief	31
Failures	29

Among the early failures, 24 were probably the result of poor selection on the basis of personality. Such patients either were considered by the surgeon before surgery as "seriously disturbed" or else have MMPIs showing elevations greater than two standard deviations from the mean on four or more scales. Of the 14 late failures, 6 had major unresolved personality problems; 4 were the result of a gradual loss of effective stimulation; 4, of uncertain cause. Thus, at least 30 of our 80 patients had such serious personality problems that we now realize they should not have been implanted.

The patient's personality thus remains a major source of concern and a major cause of failure.

Another major factor determining the success and failure of DCS is the electrode position. For the placement of 107 electrodes, we have the following results:

	EXCELLENT	FAIR	FAILURE
Epidural (outside the dura)	2	2	2
Endodural (Interdural within the dura)	1	4	8
Subdural (Extra-arachnoid beneath the dura)	12	36	40

Ideally, we should compare the electrode type in relation to the dural position; however, the small sub-classification numbers are insufficient to show significant differences.

The pre-existing disease state or physical "cause" of pain has not been of any apparent significance in determining the degree of pain relief. To some extent, we were unable to be certain of the efficacy of the DCS in some pain states, as the number of cases was small. Actually, most of our patients were failures of disc surgery!

Two iatrogenic neurologic deficits, however, did play major roles in our DCS failure statistics; all four cingulumotomy patients were considered failures; of the twelve cordotomized patients, eight were failures, three received fair relief, and one achieved excellent results. None of the cingulumotomy patients was considered emotionally stable, so it appears that this procedure, which we never recommend in cases of benign pain, has the further disadvantage of preventing other therapy from possible success. And cordotomy is no better! In cordotomized patients, DCS should be undertaken only if total pain relief is accomplished by percutaneous DCS over a 48-hour trial.

Of the 80 patients, 48 of them had complications, with a total of 77 complications between those 48. An itemization of these difficulties and the number of times they occurred is as follows:

TYPE OF COMPLICATION	FREQUENCY OF OCCURRENCE
CSF leak	16
Electrode removed	5
Prolonged pain associated with operative wounds	10

Poor localization, inadequate stimulation	12
Hematoma, incisional (minor)	5
Uncomfortable paresthesia	7
Mechanical problems, requiring re-operation, re-positioning, or repair of wire	15
Partial paraplegia	3
Infection	1
Seroma	3

Complications have been mainly mechanical. The neurologic deficits largely resulted from the placement of the older, thicker, "shielded" bipolar electrode (bipolar with three electrode contacts) in patients with small spinal canals. Almost all the patients recovered with the removal of the electrode. A new three-contact bipolar electrode may overcome this problem.

CSF (spinal fluid) leaks are a nuisance and can be prevented only by meticulous dura mater closure. When they do occur, they can be controlled within a short period by closed drainage either through the spine or in the wound itself. Seromas are uncommon with the recurrent placements and can be easily treated with drainage. Sepsis has occurred once in our series, despite routine use of prophylactic antibiotics during and after surgery. In that case, the infection became manifest one month after the implant and its seriousness was probably attenuated by the previous antibiotics. A transient increase in neurologic deficit or a reduction in position sense, motor coordination or bladder control during stimulation has been seen only in patients with considerable pre-existent deficit. Radicular pain, presumably from irritation or stimulation of the posterior roots, almost invariably clears up within three or four weeks after implantation.

Because of these various complications, I myself have not performed a DCS implant since May 1973. In fact, I believe peripheral and spinal implantations should be done only in extreme situations and only after other non-surgical approaches have been exhausted. Nevertheless, electroanalgesia has been very valuable to pain management. Certainly, TNS is by far the most widely useful, particularly since it offers safe pain relief in 80 percent of acute pain cases. Even though only 25 percent of our chronic patients achieve relief which could be termed excellent, an additional 50 percent obtain at least partial relief, so that with behavior modification they are able to bring their pain problems under control. Perhaps the major contribution of DCS has been its focusing of our work in alternative techniques for the relief of pain.

Acupuncture

We have used acupuncture in the treatment of chronic pain patients since 1967 and have found it occasionally to be of tremendous help. In about 10 percent of chronic pain patients acupuncture may make the difference between success and failure, and it may be of slight help in another 15 percent. Acupuncture is not a difficult procedure. In very simple terms, it refers to the insertion into the skin, usually, of a very fine needle. We find about a 28 gauge to be better than a 32 gauge, but a 30 gauge is also acceptable. It is a tapered needle and it has a solid core. This needle is inserted about one centimeter or sometimes as deep as two or three centimeters at strategic points all of which follow the classic meridians. However, we invariably insert our needle into a meridian in the region of the patient's pain and only go into more remote areas which might be reflexly related in the sense of Janet Travell's referral or trigger areas if therapy in the primary area does not work. There is no point trying a full explanation of the philosophy or phenomena of acupuncture. These have been widely discussed. The ideas of primordial essences of Ying and Yang and the notion of Qi, the energy of life, are quite foreign to me as well as to most other physicians.

There is, however, considerable scientific evidence that acupuncture has significant effect upon the nervous system, especially upon the autonomic nervous system. Potent somatovisceral, cutaneovisceral, viscerocutaneous, viscerosomatic, neurocutaneous, cutaneoneural, neurovisceral, visceroneural, humeroneural, and neurohumeral reflexes exist. Their functions and disorders have been extensively studied by western anatomists, neurophysiologists and endocrinologists. Although individual correlations of these pathways with appropriate acupuncture points have not been made, many acupuncture points correspond extremely well with the areas of referred pain.

In practical application of acupuncture, two factors are important. First, almost all points which are worth needling are in themselves exquisitely tender and somewhat indurated and firmer than surrounding tissue. Second, needle acupuncture in itself is painful, although the Chinese and many others have given the impression that acupuncture does not hurt. We have never found anyone in whom pain relief was accomplished if the treatment itself was not painful. Indeed, when I had a delegation of visitors from the People's Republic of China, we finally came to the conclusion that there was a semantic problem. They have dozens and dozens of words for hurt and pain, whereas we have a rather limited number. They consider the sensation of an acupuncture needle one that is "sour," and many of my patients now say, "that was very sour."

We have found several points to be most useful in the treatment of pain:

> G20, on either side of the spine at the junction of the head and neck; essentially this will put one at about C2 bilaterally; Hoku, or Large Intestine 4, in the snuff box area, a very important reflex area for arm, face, and neck pain; Bladder 26, one of the most important of all, which rather significantly overlies the sacroiliac joint.

If simple needling with twisting of the needle is not adequate, it is sometimes worthwhile to use alligator clips and connect them to one of the external electrical stimulators applying either a brief, very intense stimulation or a low-level, tingling sensation for thirty to sixty minutes. At points like the Bladder 26 point we think it is extremely important that one sometimes use an 18 or 19 gauge needle and go right down to the periosteum vigorously pounding four or five times. This is very painful but often extremely helpful in relieving the patient's pain.

Whether or not a physician wishes to use acupuncture in his program is up to him. It can be, however, extremely effective in an occasional pain patient. One such patient was a nurse who arrived in our clinic after many years of chronic, thoracic back pain and after she had had an eight-level thoracic rhizotomy. Her first acupuncture treatment in our office gave her a total relief of pain for two weeks and she was totally withdrawn from the codeine to which she had been considered addicted. When I last heard from her many months later she was receiving one acupuncture treatment each month from her pediatrician husband with good control of her pain. A patient such as this, who has tried all other modalities of therapy, including psychotherapy, without success, makes a good case for the use of acupuncture in selected pain patients.

Ice

From the beginning of our work with chronic pain, it has been obvious to us that cold is often more effective than heat, although certainly moist heat is most useful in areas of pain. We have tried repeatedly to compare the ice rubdowns which were mentioned earlier in the book with Cryogel® and Therapac® and can only come to the following conclusion: the ice rubdowns are excellent and seem to be preferred by patients, but they are cumbersome at home and very hard to administer. In areas which are irregular in contour, the Cryogel® may be useful, but it is not nearly as effective as Therapac®. Therapac® is more rigid, but delivers a measured amount of cold and is melted completely within twenty minutes so that the patient's skin is never burned by it. For home use it is often the most effective way of applying ice continuously and we recommend its use about four times a day and no more than eight times a day maximum.

Massage

Both generalized total body massage and focal massage are very useful techniques in controlling pain. Generalized massage helps create a feeling of relaxation and comfort, and is often very useful in helping patients to gain increasing mobility of joints. Focal massage is very useful especially in areas which are very hyper-sensitive and in sensory deprivation pain syndrome. Pounding massage, slapping massage, kneading or knuckling vigorously four to eight times a day may help to de-sensitize a patient who otherwise would not respond well to the total pain program.

Physical Exercise

Physical exercise is probably the most important part of our program other than autogenic training and biofeedback. First of all, we emphasize limbering exercises and the following program is used:

EXERCISES

The number of times each exercise is repeated will be determined by your physical ability to tolerate them. Begin with a minimum of 2 or 3 repetitions of each exercise and add one more each day. When you become tired or short of breath, rest, and then proceed. The exercises are to be adapted to individual needs whenever necessary. Do a complete set of exercises in consecutive order at least twice a day.

Head Rolls

Starting Position: Stand or sit erect. Allow arms to hang loosely at sides.

Action: Gently drop chin to chest and roll head to the right in a full circle. Repeat this to the left. Work up to 10 in each direction.

Purpose: Good for a stiff or aching neck or a headache.

Shoulders Up and Down

Starting Position: Stand or sit erect. Allow arms to hang loosely at sides.

Action: Bring shoulders up toward your ears as far as possible, then as far back as possible, pulling the shoulder blades together in the back. Relax to starting position. Do this in a circular motion. Keep head erect and neck straight. Work up to 20 times.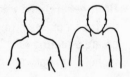

Purpose: This will loosen up the muscles of the shoulders and neck.

Wing Stretcher

Starting Position: Stand erect, elbows at shoulder height, fists clenched in front of chest or finger tips touching.

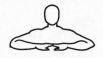

Action: Thrust elbows vigorously backward without arching back. Keep head erect, elbows at shoulder height. Return to starting position. Work up to 20 times.

Purpose: This exercise stretches the chest muscles to improve posture.

Sitting Knee Stretch

Starting Position: Sit erect on floor or mat. Legs should be straight and shoulder width apart.

Action: Bring right foot to top of left thigh with left hand. Press right knee to floor with right hand as far as possible. Release pressure and repeat. Reverse to left leg. Work up to 10 with each leg.

Purpose: Another excellent sacroiliac and hip joint exercise; helps mobility of these joints.

Body Bender

Starting Position: Stand, feet shoulder width apart, hands behind neck, fingers interlaced.

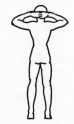

Action: Bend trunk sidewards to the right as far as possible, keeping hands behind neck. Return to starting position. Repeat to the left. Do not bend forward or backward, only to the side. Work up to 10 in each direction.

Purpose: This exercise stretches and strengthens the muscles and joints along the sides of the spine.

Hip Walks

Starting Position: Sit on floor, legs slightly separated and out straight in front of you.

Action: Walk on your seat 10 moves forward and 10 backward.

Purpose: This is good for the waist and hips.

Slow Down

Starting Position: Kneel on the floor. Hold your body from the knees up in as straight a line as possible.

Action: Lean backward from the knees as far as you can. Put both hands on heels or floor behind you for balance. Return to starting position and repeat. Work up to 20.

Purpose: This is good for the thigh muscles.

Arm Circles

Starting Position: Stand erect, arms extended sideward at shoulder height, palms up.

Action: Describe small circles backward with hands. Reverse. Turn palms down, do small circles forward. Work up to 20 of each.

Purpose: This is good for loosening up the muscles of the shoulders, shoulder blades, and upper back.

Sitting Stretch

Starting Position: Sit on floor or mat, spread legs apart, place hands on knees.

Action: Bend forward at waist, extending arms as far down legs as possible, reaching for toes. Return to starting position and repeat. Work up to 20 times.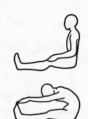

Purpose: This exercise stretches the muscles of the inner thigh.

Knee Ups

Starting Position: Stand erect, feet together, arms at sides. Lean against a wall if necessary.

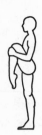

Action: Raise left knee as high as possible, grasping leg below knee and pulling knee against body. Keep back straight. Lower to starting position. Repeat with right leg. Work up to 10 of each.

Purpose: Excellent for sacroiliac joint.

Jogging in Place

Action: Run or hop in place, raising feet as high off the floor as possible. Slowly taper off speed so body function returns to normal.

Side Body Bender

Starting Position: Stand with feet slightly farther apart than shoulder width, arms loosely at sides.

Action: Step to side with right foot and point it directly outward to the right. Bend right knee. Bend body to the right, sliding right arm as far down the right leg as possible. Return to the starting position and repeat. This may be done in a "bouncing action" in which case you do not return to the starting position until you are ready to repeat to the left. Work up to 10 times with each leg.

Purpose: Good for thighs and hips.

Since we have gone to the outpatient program, because of the time involved, we have not used the swimnastics program. If you are interested in that, and it is a very excellent limbering type of exercise program, copies of the program can be obtained from the LaCrosse, Wisconsin YM-YWCA.

Finally, we think that cardiovascular strengthening exercises are appropriate and we strongly recommend *New Aerobics* and *Aerobics for Women* programs, and all patients who are not over the age of 65 or paraplegic or otherwise neurologically damaged are encouraged to begin an aerobic program within one to two months after leaving the pain rehabilitation program. Then within 16 weeks they should have achieved their maximum cardiovascular level and should remain at that.

CHAPTER IX
Biogenics

In addition to curing himself of his old game-playing habits and instilling instead patterns of healthy behavior, the pain patient needs to come to terms with his emotions which are at least a contributing factor to his pain and may very well be the prime cause in some cases. He needs to realize that in terms of creating and perpetuating pain and illness, he may be his own enemy. But once he recognizes that the functioning of his body—whether for good or ill health—is under his volition, those tables can be turned; he can, then, through autogenic training and biofeedback assist in working his own "cure"—pain management through self-regulation.

As a method of acquiring mind and body self-regulation, autogenic training was developed in the 1920s in Germany by Johannes H. Schultz who believed that voluntary and predictable control of the body could be attained by programming it to develop heavy and warm extremities, a warm abdomen, a calm and regular heartbeat, relaxed respiration and a cool forehead. Autogenic training, actually then, is sensory biofeedback.

Actually, the practice dates back even further than that in control of physiological processes through long practice of particular mental disciplines. Indeed, early in this century two related techniques were developed. In 1910, Emil Coué, a French pharmacist, elaborated his system of autosuggestion, a simple general approach to psychosomatic attunement, "Every day, in every way, I am getting better and better." Thousands of patients were successfully treated with this technique. Less than two decades later, a Chicago physician, Edmund Jacobson, introduced "progessive relaxation." His technique, he insisted, had nothing to do with "suggestion or autosuggestion." But most psychophysiologic symptoms were reported to be markedly improved by the regular practice of simple deep relaxation. Spastic colon, globus hystericus, chronic insomnia, compulsion neuroses, phobias, neurasthenia, anxiety neurosis, compulsive tics, depression (even manic depressives), hyperthyroidism, stuttering and stammering, etc., all benefitted.

In 1959, Maharishi Mahesh Yogi introduced Transcendental Meditation® to the Western world. This approach is much more mystical and metaphysical but aside from the cult-like aspect of being initiated by a personal secret word, it primarily teaches passive, dispassionate relaxation. Extensive work has demonstrated its effectiveness in a wide variety of psychophysiologic symptoms. However, it has not been proven of value in the desperate chronic pain patient, and it has led to some cases of catatonia as it is rather passive.

Despite the tremendous data behind autogenic training, the most scientific and rigidly studied of these psychophysiologic approaches, American physicians have largely ignored it. Of about 3,000 publications related to autogenic training, less than 300 are in English and most of the English articles are written by the Japanese!

The idea of autogenic training did not really catch on in this country until biofeedback, which is the mechanical device for measuring and monitoring simple physiologic activities, was developed in 1961. By observing the evidence of his ability to manage his body's activities (for instance, a patient can see for himself that it is possible for him to raise or lower his skin temperature) the patient trains himself to control actions of his body which he had previously thought tbxinvoluntary: his heartbeat, his breathing, his temperature, and, importantly for our patients, his pain. As a part of teaching the patient to control his autonomic nervous system which regulates the internal organs, the goal of all autogenic methods is harmonious limbic-hypothalamic, that is emotional, balance, To acquire that regulation or attunement, the patient needs to learn to sublimate his negative emotions, not to suppress them, but to overcome feelings of paranoia, anger, hatred, frustration, self-pity and depression which are so often a part of the make-up of the chronic pain sufferer. Because emotional stress puts a strain on the body as well, the purpose of autogenics and biofeedback training is to evoke changes opposite to that of stress for both therapeutic and preventive reasons.

We have been surprised by the warm reception many of our patients give the ideas and techniques of autogenics and biofeedback and also the rapidity with which they have been able to develop these procedures for their benefit. However, we do run into some skeptics. Approaching such patients with the idea that habits, attitudes, and emotions may be part of their problem can be difficult to do, because some patients quickly become defensive; however, if they are to profit from autogenic training, it is essential that they know how much wear and tear negative emotions can have on their bodies and the benefits that they as pain patients, and indeed as people, can reap if they get in touch with their feelings and their bodies' actions and reactions. When I tell my patients that from 60 to 85 percent of all physical symptoms are psychosomatic (i.e. induced by emotional stress) or at least have a psychosomatic component, that comment raises a few hackles; to some people it means only one thing: their pain is all "in the head" and they are—in layman's terms—"nuts." And for those who have taken the advice to seek psychiatric help for their pain problems—very expensive, lengthy, and most likely, unfruitful advice—such a remark only adds insult to injury! Deeply ingrained in their thinking is the idea that talking of the emotional and mental influences of their pain is the same as admitting fakery: somehow, to their way of thinking, if the pain is "real," then the emotions or the mind did not cause it, nor can they effect a cure.

Actually, the medical profession has encouraged this misconception with a couple of its own. First, the idea that the mind and body are separate entities: psychiatrists are supposed to deal with one entity and physicians the other. But the mind and body are in fact inseparable and for that reason effective treatment has to include both. Yet, while even medical students know that a large percentage of illness is psychosomatic, most doctors do not deal with illness as a psychosomatic problem; and, of course, the idea of psychosomatic *health* is practically unheard of! The premises of psychic origin for good and ill health are neither understood very well nor put into effect; rather than being a part of every doctor's province, psychosomatic illness is in fact considered a specialty, or, by default, is treated psychiatrically. Indeed, medical students are not taught any techniques for treating emotion-induced illness. Rather, they learn surgical or pharmaceutical manipulation of the end organ symptom. Typically, when a doctor does suspect that a certain illness, say an ulcer, has been induced by emotional stress, he believes he can treat the physical ulcer; and then the rest of the problem, the emotional half, can be turned over to a psychiatrist. This two-part approach is, of course, nonsensical since it rests on the false assumption that there is a dichotomy of mind and body.

But medical research in the last 25 years has encouraged this assumption. Symptoms and organs have been dissected physiologically, microsurgically, and sub-microscopically and chemically without cross-correlation with the neural and/or emotional impulses affecting disease. Independently, however, extensive investigation of the nervous systems has confirmed the possibility that almost every conceivable pathological process can be produced by some sort of brain or nervous stimulation.

Finally, the idea that the patient can and ought to manage, at least in part, his own pain or illness, flies in the face of traditional medical thinking. The whole thing smacks too much of self-treatment (which is justifiably frowned upon in cases of self-diagnosis or self-administration of medication) or worse yet, it sounds a lot like the bugbear of the medical profession, faith healing! Consequently, even though there is evidence proving its effectiveness, autogenics is often seen, at most, as the very last resort for unresponsive cases. It is not surprising then that some patients have come to expect to be passively treated and not to initiate any sort of self-control. Unfortunately, many of them come with the idea that since the pain is in their bodies, that is where they want their therapy to be; and as indicated, some of those therapeutic methods can have disastrous results.

To the patients who may be resistant to the idea of autogenics, we try to make it clear as possible that we are not suggesting that their pain—or for that matter, any of their physical maladies—are imaginary. Nor do we want to imply that they are willful schemers. Rather, we try to define with them, through lectures and conferences, which physical and emotional factors are contributing and influencing that pain. Since as part of our operant conditioning program we discourage them from cataloging their ailments and belaboring how difficult it is to be in pain, our conferences can be more rational and less hysterical. If nothing else, by refusing to be a wailing wall for my patients, I am able to save the time for more constructive conferences about their problems and the contributing factors.

A majority of symptoms—pain included—are directly caused by or at least aggravated by unresolved emotional stress. The attitude of the patient at the time of an emotional insult determines whether a symptom will develop and where the symptom will be felt. In general some part of the body will react to most emotional stress. If the stress is persistent, chronic, then symptoms may gradually lead to actual physical disturbance, through prolonged and/or intense physiologic change.

Whenever someone is alerted to a physical danger, his heart beats rapidly (or it may even slow to the point of death), he gets cold and sweaty, his breathing becomes heavy, he may get diarrhea, or conversely, his intestines may suddenly cease functioning, and he may have bladder spasms. No one would argue that these physical symptoms are simply figments of the imagination; they are, rather, very real, physical manifestations of an emotion: fear. Less apparent, but still verifiable, fright can also cause the serum cortisone and the adrenaline levels to soar and numerous other chemical changes to take place as well.

The case of fright in reaction to a real danger offers the perfect illustration of emotions being translated into effects upon the body. Once the danger is over, however, the fear usually subsides and the body most likely will return to normal functioning. But, man often reacts to threats and signs of danger as strongly as he does to actual physical danger; indeed, sometimes imagined or emotional threats can be far more harmful to him than palpable danger because the stress itself may cause more harm to his body than the danger which may or may not in fact materialize. And many aspects of life can be a source of this stress: love, marriage, children, work, money, retirement, even a promotion, death of a loved one, loss of a job, war, etc. Other, more obviously traumatic events are not necessarily more capable of producing stress than the everyday, seemingly innocuous elements of life such as marriage or a career. In fact, this type of tension may be even more insidious than, say, a good scare because it is an on-going, day-in day-out kind of stress. Of course, certain stress such as anger may be a much greater disturbance at some times than at others. If an individual has had insufficient sleep, for instance, he may get upset with the noise his children normally make, whereas if everything else were stable, he might even join them in their play. A lot of different elements—education, family background, intelligence, talents, prejudices, and relationships with parents, siblings, spouse and superiors—are contributing factors which influence how a person reacts to a given emotional stimulus. But, for whatever reasons, the important fact is that emotional stress wreaks havoc with the body; the list of physical illness so induced is both long and impressive.

There are a number of processes which lead to disease, processes known to be strongly influenced by psychosomatic stresses. Illness or dis-ease may be symptomatic, physical, chemical, electrical, emotional, or combinations of all these. Diseases are generally divided into the following five categories: (1) congenital, (2) traumatic,(3) neoplastic, (4) infectious, and (5) degenerative—trophic, immunologic, vascular, hormonal, emotional, and chemical balance influence all of these.

There is no proof that the usual physical deformities considered congenital are psychosomatic. Some psychiatrists, however, have theorized that many mental disorders begin in *utero;* the physical development of the fetus is, of course, strongly influenced by the mother's physical health, her diet and drug intake, including cigarette smoking, influences which affect and are affected by her emotional health.

Acute trauma, on the other hand, is probably more accurately typed psychosomatic. Not every trauma is, of course, self-caused, but many people who are accident prone and have repeated mishaps need to come to grips with their self-destructive bent. Since 75 percent of all accidents occur on "critical" days in the biorhythm and are a result of care-less-ness, *not caring,* then the psychologic aspects of trauma are nonetheless real! In such cases, obviously, treatment must first be aimed at the physical problems created by the accident, but some effort should also be directed to personality problems. Since many chronic pain patients are suffering as the result of injuries received in accidents such as falls or traffic collisions, counseling, operant conditioning and autogenic training are necessary to prevent recurrent injuries. Case histories on such patients reveal that rarely is a single incident the "cause" of their pain; more likely, one mishap is followed by another, and another. Sometimes, a patient may find his pain temporarily relieved by a certain therapy only to re-injure himself. This is one of the reasons I am convinced that behavior modification is an essential part of the patient's cure.

In cases of neoplasia, i.e. tumor growth, a number of psychological studies have suggested a strong relation between personality and cancer. Diet, immune-reaction, drugs, pollutants, and toxins, smoking, hormones, smog, viruses—all are of considerable importance and ultimately must interact to make one "cancer-prone." Nevertheless, it may be that a basic emotional upset is essential for these physical factors to induce malignant alterations. Once the cancer has started, its time course may be influenced by alterations in any and/or all of the basic factors which are known to "cause" cancer. These factors include emotions—which may explain how faith healing has been able to effect verifiable cancer remissions.

All individuals are exposed to a great many and a variety of infectious agents. Some will, as a result, become ill and some of those will die. Diet and general over-all health undoubtedly influence the relative activities of each individual's immune abilities; for instance, even though a majority of Americans have antibodies to the hepatitis virus, few have active, acute hepatitis. It is not unreasonable to assume that emotional balance can help keep the immune mechanisms working properly. Once active infections develop, patients vary tremendously in their reactions: they develop immunities—either slowly or rapidly—some recover and some die. To these ends, they are aided, hindered or harmed by a variety of therapies; in appropriate cases, antibiotics are statistically the most effective, but, again, faith healing cannot be ruled out as useless since it may restore the emotional balance necessary to develop immunity. Anyhow, it has been known to work.

The remaining bulk of diseases—degenerative, trophic, immunologic, vascular, hormonal, and emotional—are obviously influenced by heredity, diet, the immune reaction, toxins, etc. Interestingly, the mental disorders, e.g. the psychoses such as schizophrenia, ordinarily thought to be totally psychiatric may have as the basic inciting agent a relatively simple chemical or electrical disorder in the brain. On the other side of the coin, those diseases customarily thought to be physical disorders are almost invariably intertwined with recognized emotional stress and instability. Among other things, all of this suggests that our traditional medical notions, concerning which diseases are physical and which are mental, need drastic reworking.

Stress most often manifests itself as pain since pain and anxiety are linked: a high level of anxiety can lower one's pain tolerance and increase his subjective response to pain, and pain, in turn, can also produce or increase anxiety. Of course, all pain sensations that come from any of the internal organs are conducted to the brain through the autonomic nervous system. Outside the body's cavities and the spinal canal, the autonomic nervous system reaches the arms and legs not by its own separate nerve trunk but on the coattails of the blood vessels where its primary function is to control the circulation of the blood. Temperature biofeedback offers the best chance to alter these functions. Indeed, extensive reports indicate that temperature and EMG biofeedback are effective in about 80 percent of patients suffering from headache pain.

Actually, the most common symptom known to man, headache, often comes from muscle tension: sustained contraction of neck muscles brought on by emotional tenseness. Muscles throughout the body, representing the greatest bulk of tissue, are responsible also for a majority of symptoms. Backaches, leg and arm pains are often due to muscle tension—which is appropriately called *armoring* by the great psychiatrist Wilhelm Reich—muscle tension that is brought on by dissatisfaction, anger, resentment, fear, or restrained emotions of almost any type.

Even a disease such as glaucoma may be the result of emotionally induced muscle tension, since even some healthy individuals develop increased eye pressure when confronted by conflict. Many eye symptoms—conjunctivitus, for one, even blindness—have been found to be caused by depression, fear and guilt. And glaucoma has been reduced by biofeedback training, using ocular pressure and mental programming.

Tension of the diaphragm and abdominal muscles affected by emotional stress contributes to high blood pressure and a variety of intra-abdominal symptoms. For one, spasm—or tension of urinary bladder muscles—is often associated with anger and resentment, usually suppressed. In individuals under steady emotional stress, constipation is often a problem; or it may be diarrhea; or alternating diarrhea and constipation, a condition known as spastic colon. There may be gallbladder problems, such as gallstones or kidney stones. Women may have menstrual irregularities or difficulties in becoming pregnant, and problems of sexual potency may result in men.

Asthma, allergies, rashes and skin problems are often evidence of the autonomic system's imbalance. Even illnesses like flu and colds have been significantly related to emotional turmoil, such sickness most frequently occurring at times of acute stress or in those who have the worst life-adjustment problems. Indeed, simple fatigue and listlessness have their beginnings in various emotions.

Other illnesses—some of them a lot more serious—are similarly generated by emotional imbalance. If a person gets angry enough and suppresses it long enough, he can get a peptic ulcer. And, if that ruptures, or a blood vessel ruptures, it is possible that he could bleed to death or die of peritonitis—a potentially fatal physical problem which began as an imbalance of emotions. People can also die of ulcerative colitis which is another perfect illustration of the most serious kind of emotional influence on the colon. In hyptertension which brings with it the possibility of heart attack or stroke, emotions and personality are considered contributing factors. It may even be possible to correlate specific emotions and attitudes with specific diseases.

Certain personality patterns have, in fact, been shown to correlate with particular illnesses. Cancer patients very often are passive people who do not square themselves off against the aggravations of life; apparently, their immune mechanisms do no better against the incursions of malignant cells. And often they are people who generally endure, silently, the inevitable insults of life without outwardly expressing the anger or unhappiness they no doubt feel. In addition, they are often people who have suffered some major loss—like the death of a loved one, or divorce—within eighteen months to two years before the onset of the disease. Another case in point is the hypertensive person who is presumably in the greatest danger of developing coronary heart disease. His personality pattern: He is a chronic, frenetic worker, who undertakes everything seriously and competitively. He perhaps has nervous habits and is often impatient with and aggressive to those around him—and underneath it all, he has a sense of guilt if he is not up and doing. This personality has been labeled *type A* but it is likely to earn a fat zero in life expectancy!

Since all of these diseases are truly self-destructive processes, the ideal treatment would involve reprogramming the patient's emotional and physical make-up in order to avoid the inevitable illness. In some cases, there may not be time, of course, and surgery and drugs, often an unfortunate choice, are the only sensible approach. If a peptic ulcer, for instance, is hemorrhaging or on the verge of doing so, the treatment must be immediate. There is no time then to deal with causes. But, if those causes are not also dealt with, the ulcer will most likely recur. Psychiatrists have long known that if one psychosomatic symptom is erased without getting at the causes for the symptom, another will surely take its place or another kind of autonomic dysfunction will occur.

Then too, not all stress is emotional. Physiological changes can also be brought on, for instance, by the ingestion of drugs. Even the commonplace aspirin can eat a hole in a person's stomach lining, if that person takes enough of it. And things like cigarettes and caffeine, whether in coffee or cola drinks, can act adversely upon the body's chemistry Other factors, which are largely outside the individual's control—like environmental pollutants, or heredity—also go into the creation of disease.

It is the autonomic nervous system which governs the body physiology, the inner organs that generally function below the conscious level; it regulates the activities of these structures such as respiration, blood pressure, circulation, heart beat, digestion, body temperature, metabolism, sweating, the secretion of certain endocrine glands, etc. In other words, the autonomic nervous system is what makes the body run. It has long been believed that the inner organs and their activities are not under volitional control, but there is evidence that the autonomic nervous system can be brought under voluntary control or self-regulation through training techniques.

The autonomic nervous system, in turn, is managed by the hypothalamus, the master switch in the brain that regulates all other inner physiology. The hypothalamus is surrounded by the limbic system—the emotional center of the brain—and has connections with it; and it is through the limbic system's influence on the hypothalamus that emotional disturbances are transferred to the body. Conversely, by avoiding emotional excesses, it is possible to balance the hypothalamus and the autonomic nervous system. It has been shown experimentally in animals that electrical stimulation of certain parts of the hypothalamus can drive the blood pressure up to the point of stroke or create peptic ulceration within hours. The limbic system can as easily, although not as quickly, get out of tune through emotional stress and the result is hardening of the arteries, peptic ulcer, rheumatoid arthritis, or a host of other psychosomatic symptoms—*including, most commonly, pain.* The purpose of autogenic and biofeedback training is to get the limbic and the autonomic nervous systems, that is the emotional and the somatic functions, balanced in order to prevent or overcome psychophysiologic problems. It is also possible to realign these two systems through religious faith or spiritual meditation or self-hypnosis or even art and music. Although I do not want to deny the effectiveness of these methods, they are not acceptable to everyone; autogenics, I believe, is more agreeable to more people. Ideally, however, we would like to expose our patients to all methods and then let each one decide which of the methods is acceptable, which he can live with and which he will practice for the rest of his life.

Normally, the brain has a certain rate of rhythmic electrical activity measured in pulses or cycles per second. The *beta* state of mind of 14 to 22 pulses per second is that of wide-awake awareness when the mind is conscious of what is outside it. The *alpha* state of 8 to 13 cycles per second usually occurs during close, intent concentration when the mind is not so susceptible to distraction. The *theta* state, which is 4 to 7 cycles, occurs when the mind becomes even more withdrawn from what is happening externally. More of what we call creativity occurs during this reverie when the artist or the scientist or whoever is so intent on creating a new work or a new idea that he is oblivious to his surroundings.

Individuals who are deeply hypnotized are usually in a *theta* state. If the brain gears down even further and is pulsing from one to three sycles per second, it is in a *delta* state and sleep occurs. In both the *theta* and the *alpha* states, significant distress is not very likely, because stress, whether it is emotional or physical, is an alerting mechanism which accelerates the brain's activities up into the *beta* state. *If a person can purposefully put himself back down into* alpha *or* theta *states and remain there, he can suppress his pain.*

It is also possible to control bleeding. It has been demonstrated that if surgery is done under hypnosis (the brain is in the *theta* state) there is much less blood loss than under ordinary anesthesia, because anesthesia increases venous pressure and decreases proper breathing, and, without it, there is naturally less bleeding. But, in addition, individuals have such good control over their autonomic nervous system functions they can actually regulate their blood vessels.

However, it is possible to program the mind to slow down its electrical activity without hypnosis. It is possible through breathing exercises, relaxation and concentration to drop down to *theta* and *alpha* states. And, most importantly, cultivating the ability to decrease the full-speed activity of the brain also normalizes and regulates body functions of all sorts: the heartbeat becomes calm and regular, the metabolic rate goes down; the respiration is slow and even, and each of the internal organs operates with quiet ease. During this state, the body can be mentally programmed, and instructions given to it will be carried out; emotions as well can be examined and if found unacceptable, they can be regulated into acceptable ones. Getting down to the *alpha* or *theta* states or to fall asleep requires that either there is total concentration on a single thing or on nothing at all. The most time-honored techniques of dropping to the *alpha* state requires voluntary regulation of breathing. The normal rate of breathing of sixteen to twenty times per minute is actually inefficient, too rapid really to fill the lungs. Slowing the rate to about four per minute and breathing deeply and completely is one of the quickest ways of entering a more relaxed state of mind.

The purpose of both autogenic and biofeedback training (biogenics) is to balance and alter—beneficially—body function through mental concentration. Much more study remains to be done verifying how statistically successful this method of maintaining good health is and what factors go into determining its effectiveness, but preliminary studies indicate it can be very effective. In a pilot study done on migraine and tension headaches, it was found that if a patient is able to increase the blood flow to his hands within two minutes of the onset of a headache—which would be evidenced by a 10° F. increase in his hand temperature—he could stave off an impending attack. Another study testing the effectiveness of electromyographic (EMG) feedback in reducing intensity and frequency of tension headache found that if subjects were given incorrect data indicating that muscles were relaxed when they were not in fact, the pattern of frequency and intensity did not differ from that without feedback at all. However, accurate feedback was able to reduce the number and the intensity of such headaches.

Although the idea that cancer is a psychosomatic disease may be too far-fetched for some, Dr. Carl Simonton is convinced otherwise. He noticed that a certaim small percentage of cancer patients responded to treatment much more readily and unexpectedly than others to the point that such cases actually defied medical prognoses. In talking with these patients he found consistently that they were people with positive attitudes who simply refused to die. On the other hand, those patients who did not respond to treatment, in spite of their expressed wishes to continue living, were found to be depressed and indifferent to life, perhaps on some level even wishing to die, as Freud emphasized. That the mind determines the body's immune response or resistance, is now medically proven; and, according to Dr. Simonton, whether a patient wants to live or wants to die determines whether or not his body will resist the growth of cancerous cells. To mobilize the mind's power in order that it might prod the body's resistance, he used mental balancing techniques in which the patient completely relaxed his body and envisioned himself becoming well, visualizing the immune mechanisms of his body going to work and the medical therapy effectively combating the milignant cells. In his study of 152 patients, Dr. Simonton found that those patients who were cooperative in their treatment—which involved, usually, radiation but also chemotherapy and surgery as well as psychotherapy and meditation—and enthusiastic about getting well, did in fact show a marked relief of their symptoms. Further study has indicated similar results.

In another report, clinical experience indicates that various somatic symptoms such as chronic headache, Raynaud's disease, vascular hypertension, weakness, palpitation, and fatigue, disappeared readily with biofeedback training; and, as a beneficial side effect, these patients reported that they felt more confident and capable of functioning in relation to themselves and other people. Essential hypertension, that is elevated blood pressure without a demonstrable cause, might be controlled since it has been shown that a person can modify his systolic pressure if given feedback data. In short, it appears that 80 percent of *all* symptoms are amenable to biogenic training.

Our biogenic training program is comprised of a series of lectures which deal with our philosophy of pain management and the role that mental attitudes—both positive and negative—can play in producing health and ill-health; and a series of mental exercises in which the patient practices reducing the stress on his body and programming it to be pain- and sickness-free.

There are various exercises which we try with our patients allowing them to discover and decide for themselves which are most effective in relieving their pain symptoms or in giving them feelings of well-being. When they leave the center, they are instructed to continue practicing with exercises they themselves choose and which we have taped for them. Such practice up to ten or twelve hours a day at first may be necessary.

When the patient learns to relax totally, it is essential for him to find a comfortable position which, for most people, means lying flat with hands and legs uncrossed; eventually, however, relaxation should be possible in any position.

Each practice session begins with the directions to breathe deeply and to relax. Deep breathing shifts the autonomic nervous system into low gear, so that it functions easily and without stress. Relaxation is the key to all the exercises because it allows the patient to drop down to the *alpha* state, to be undistracted by external activity and by stressful thoughts and emotions. Often when our patients first try total relaxation—something they almost never do except in sleep—they doze off. But they soon learn that it is possible to remain completely alert while experiencing this really delightful feeling. Once they have reached that point of relaxed awareness, it is possible for them to go within themselves objectively without external influences, to program their body physiology by repeating appropriate suggestions to it and by visualizing the desired results.

One basic exercise for pain relief is as follows:

Now relax, close your eyes, take a deep breath and repeat mentally to yourself each sentence after I say it.

My arms and legs are heavy and warm. (6 times)

My heartbeat is calm and regular. (6 times)

My body breathes itself. (6 times)

My abdomen is warm. (6 times)

My forehead is cool. (6 times)

My mind is quiet and still. (3 times)

My mind is quiet and happy. (3 times)

I am at peace.

I feel my feet expanding lightly and pleasantly by 1 inch. (2 times)

My feet are now expanding lightly and pleasantly by 12 inches. (2 times)

The pleasant 12-inch expansion is spreading throughout all the parts of my legs. (2 times)

My abdomen, buttocks, and back are expanding 12 inches lightly and pleasantly. (2 times)

My chest is expanding 12 inches pleasantly and lightly. (2 times)

My arms are expanding 12 inches lightly and pleasantly. (2 times)

My neck and head are joining in the 12 inches of expansion. (2 times)

My entire body is relaxed, expanded and comfortable. (6 times)

My mind is quiet and still. (2 times)

I withdraw my mind from my physical surroundings. (2 times)

I am free of pain and all other sensations. (2 times)

My body is safe and comfortable. (6 times)

My mind is quiet and happy. (2 times)

I am that I am. (pause 2 minutes)

Each time I practice this exercise my body becomes more and more comfortable. And I carry this comfort with me to my normal awareness. As I prepare to return to my normal awareness I will bring with me the ideal comfort which I have created in my focused concentration. As I open my eyes, I take a deep comfortable breath and a big comfortable stretch.

As the patient practices biogenic training—and for pain that means from four to twelve hours per day—he gradually learns to enter an altered state of feeling and awareness, in which no body sensations are felt but in which his mind is incredibly alert; and he is perfectly, ideally conscious, seemingly capable of coming up with the answers to any questions. If his EEG is being recorded at this time his brain is pulsing electrically in a slow, steady *alpha* or *theta* rhythm. Repeated verbal and visual programming in this state of body-mind harmony gradually produces greater and greater freedom from pain, a comfort which can be carried over into the normal states of activity for longer periods of time. Repeated practice is essential and *it may require six to ten months of practice before it is possible to achieve consistent pain relief.*

There are other exercises our patients try, each of them intending to counteract the effects of emotional stress upon the body. The following exercises illustrate:

SELF-LOVE EXERCISE

Relax. Close your eyes. Take a deep breath and relax. Now repeat after me each phrase. (Pause 15 seconds after each.)

My arms and legs are heavy and warm. (3 times)

My heartbeat is calm and regular. (3 times)

My body breathes itself. (3 times)

My abdomen is warm. (3 times)

My forehead is cool. (3 times)

My mind is quiet and still. (3 times)

I am at peace.

I am very happy. (4 times)

I succeed in my greatest desires. (4 times)

Every day in every way I am becoming more and more healthy. (4 times)

I have a very healthy and happy mind. (4 times)

I have a very healthy and loving mind. (4 times)

I am building a beautifully functioning body and mind. (4 times)

I love and appreciate all my excellent abilities. (4 times)

I know that my innermost being is magnificent, wise, and loving. (4 times)

I love and appreciate the universal life force which sustains me. (4 times)

Each time I practice these exercises, I gain more of my desires.

Every day in every way I am becoming more and more healthy.

Now as I prepare to return to my normal awareness, I feel myself bringing with me the health, happiness, comfort, and love I feel and see. I take another deep breath—eyes open —wide open—feeling happy and refreshed, feeling the energy flowing into all parts of my body.

EMIL COUÉ SPECIAL EXERCISE

Relax. Assume your most comfortable possible position. Close your eyes. Take a deep breath and repeat to yourself each sentence in all the pauses.

(Pause 15 seconds after each sentence throughout)

Every day in every way I am getting better and better.
Every day in every way I am getting better and better.
Every day in every way I am getting better and better.
Every day in every way I am getting better and better.
Every day in every way I am getting better and better.

Every day in every way I am becoming more and more healthy.
Every day in every way I am becoming more and more healthy.
Every day in every way I am becoming more and more healthy.
Every day in every way I am becoming more and more healthy.
Every day in every way I am becoming more and more healthy.

I am free of all outside forces.
I am free of all outside forces.

I use my own consciousness to be free of all outside forces.
I use my own consciousness to be free of all outside forces.

I have everything within myself to enjoy every minute of every day.
I have everything within myself to enjoy every minute of every day.

I am always responsible for my thoughts and actions.
I am always responsible for my thoughts and actions.

I accept myself completely here and now.
I accept myself completely here and now.

I feel loving compassion for all other human beings.
I feel loving compassion for all other human beings.

I am free of all outside forces.
I am free of all outside forces.

I am attuned to my highest spiritual goals.
I am attuned to my highest spiritual goals.

I am filled with loving kindness.
I am filled with loving kindness.

I love freely and openly.
I love freely and openly.

Every day in every way I am getting better and better.
Every day in every way I am getting better and better.
Every day in every way I am getting better and better.
Every day in every way I am getting better and better.
Every day in every way I am getting better and better.
Every day in every way I am getting better and better.
Every day in every way I am getting better and better.
Every day in every way I am getting better and better.

Every day in every way I am becoming more and more healthy.
Every day in every way I am becoming more and more healthy.
Every day in every way I am becoming more and more healthy.

My arms and legs are heavy and warm.
My arms and legs are heavy and warm.
My arms and legs are heavy and warm.

My heartbeat is calm and regular.
My heartbeat is calm and regular.
My heartbeat is calm and regular.

My body breathes itself freely and comfortably.
My body breathes itself freely and comfortably.
My body breathes itself freely and comfortably.

My abdomen is warm.
My abdomen is warm.
My abdomen is warm.

My forehead is cool.
My forehead is cool.
My forehead is cool.

My mind is quiet and still.
My mind is quiet and still.
My mind is quiet and still.

I am relaxed and comfortable.
I am relaxed and comfortable.
I am relaxed and comfortable.

Every day in every way I am getting better and better.
Every day in every way I am getting better and better.
Every day in every way I am getting better and better.

I take another deep breath and as I open my eyes I stretch comfortably, feeling all the parts of my body filled with energy.

In each of the exercises the patient relaxes his body and repeats directions given by the instructor, thus programming his body to react to directions from his mind. In the hand levitation exercises, the patient concentrates on one of his hands, which is positioned by his side, and he focuses on its presence and the blood flowing to it, all the while visualizing it resting on his forehead. Many patients are surprised to find that one of their hands does indeed move up to their foreheads, proving how readily the body does respond to directions. Other exercises instruct the patient to tune in his body. The multi-awareness exercises direct the body to relax and expand while the patient visualizes, and experiences, peaceful imagery.

In the physiologic exercises, the patient concentrates on and examines mentally the organs and members of his body while at the same time feeling the heartbeat transmitted into these parts which then become warm and relaxed. Simultaneously, he concentrates on feelings of happiness and emotional warmth. Another, the pulse localization exercise, similarly calls attention to the part of the body focusing on the warming pulses of the heartbeat in each. A squirming exercise offers a way of relaxing both mind and body, directing the patient to tense and then relax certain muscles while envisoning certain colors. In the breathing exercise, the patient concentrates on and regulates his respiration, deepening his breathing and slowing it down to about four breaths per minute. In an exercise concentrating on self-image, the patient visualizes changing his body into that of another family member before returning to his own real image of perfect health.

Other exercises concentrate on particular problems like overweight or insomnia, attempting to program the body to be satisfied with less food, to relax enough to sleep, to reduce alcohol intake, or to stop smoking.

Biofeedback training involves a therapeutic machine, a teaching device which helps the patient learn to modify and control certain physiologic functions and states of mind which have been previously believed not subject to voluntary control. Like autogenics, it is based on the assumption that if the patient can be taught to control his internal state, he can also be taught to modify his pain, or, for that matter, any illnesses which are psychosomatic. Once he produces apparent change in his autonomic nervous system—which is made manifest by the feedback of the machine—he becomes aware that malfunctioning of his body is also self-produced. Biofeedback reinforces the idea that many physical symptoms do not just happen; in fact the majority of symptoms are either directly caused by or at least aggravated by unresolved stress.

There are various types of biofeedback training: brainwave or *alpha* training in which one learns to modify his brain wave output; temperature biofeedback instruction, in which the patient learns to raise or lower the skin temperature of a portion of the body; EMG (electromyogram) training, in which one learns to relax certain muscles more effectively. Many other types of biofeedback training are now being developed, or proposed, for control of almost any physiologic activity. The training is done with a battery-driven electronic machine which is calibrated to pick up extremely small physiological, electrical, or chemical changes as they take place. These minute changes (often as tiny as *one millionth* of a volt) are converted to either visual or auditory signals the patient can recognize which allow him to know immediately when changes occur. The functions monitored are those in which a person is not usually able to detect changes, such as the number of *alpha* brain waves the brain is producing from moment to moment. Thus, "biofeedback" feeds back to the patient signals showing changes in one of the biological functions.

Over a period of days (or sometimes weeks), using the biofeedback machine for about sixty minutes a day, the patient begins to learn to modify and later to control (self-regulate) the particular function he is monitoring. The machines themselves *do not* exert *any* form of control; they only relay the message of what the patient himself is altering. Once the patient becomes aware of what's going on inside his body, which is what the machine tells him, he can begin to associate those changes in body function with subtle changes in his conscious feelings—his subjective awareness. He may notice feelings of warmth, of contentment or solitude, of relaxation (sensory biofeedback), for instance, which occur when the physical biofeedback machine tells him he is producing the desirable change in his body.

With continued practice in biofeedback training, one's *appreciation* of subjective feelings certainly is enhanced. Eventually, the patient finds that he can anticipate the biofeedback signals and has to depend less and less on the machine to know when, for example, he is producing steady *alpha* waves or is changing the temperature of some part of his body. After the patient finds he is able to use his own awareness and feelings to tell him his internal functions (sensory biofeedback or autogenics), he no longer needs an external device to feed external signals back to him. Once that point has been reached, he has learned to use more effectively another portion of his body, a portion which had been there all the time but which he had never before used or appreciated.

The possibilities for what biogenic training can do for anyone, pain patients in particular, are endless. For those who find it difficult to relax, or to stop feeling worried, tense, or frustrated about something in their lives—and it is the inability to relax and stop worrying which aggravates and intensifies pain—the technique offers a saner, safer solution than most: It is no longer necessary for the patient to take a tranquilizer or a drink or to rely on mind-blowing, pain-killing drugs, or to "talk out" his problems with someone else. If nothing else, he can save considerable money and time and, at the same time, avoid the inevitable problems that drugs and alcohol create, not to mention the enhanced self-confidence and independence he can achieve.

To the best of our knowledge, biogenics has no real adverse side effects, which is more than can be said about a lot of other therapeutic methods. However, it is not yet widely used because, for one thing, the idea itself is relatively new, and newer models and methods are still emerging from the laboratory. Consequently, biogenics hasn't really had the time yet to be used on any large scale. Also, the machines have been (and still are) prohibitively expensive for individual doctors or patients to purchase. These problems will, no doubt, be solved in a matter of time. What will be more difficult to deal with is our conditioned expectation that immediate and lasting relief comes in the form of a pill, an operation, or some therapeutic method which is worked upon us. Ideas change slowly, as a rule, so it may take some time before biogenics is accepted, particularly since it requires that the patient himself work at reprogramming his body, and since the effects are not instantaneous.

Patients with *active* asthma, high blood pressure and peptic ulcer should begin biogenics under careful physician supervision, as these aggressive psychophysiologic disturbances may stubbornly worsen during the early days of biogenic training.

Our greatest success in controlling pain with biogenics has been in cases of paraplegic pain syndrome: Six out of seven such patients have gained total or near total relief. The last one refused even to try the approach, as she was primarily concerned with her inability to walk and was upset that we did not have her physically picked up and moved about in a semblance of walking. On the other hand, after seven years of agony, one 60-year-old paraplegic gained pain relief after only forty-eight hours of beginning *alpha* training, which seemed the best technique for this particular pain problem.

We, of course, emphasize the importance of progressive physical exercise to our other patients, and for that reason, among others, it is more difficult to define the exact role that autogenics and/or biofeedback played in their pain relief. In addition, all our patients have tried electrical stimulation and about one-fourth of them have had facet rhizotomies. However, in spite of the different factors that may have gone into achieving pain control, we have found that 80 percent of our patients who practice biogenics at home for six months or more, report that their pain relief has been at least 50 percent and in some cases as high as 100 percent. This actually turns out to be 63 percent of patients who *remain* improved. Most of the others just fail to practice.

But regardless of the degree of pain relief, we have found most of our patients to be open-minded, even enthusiastic about accepting responsibility for controlling their pain. Once the idea of self-regulation and biofeedback has been introduced to them, they are not adverse to being taught to help themselves —physically and mentally—and to take charge of how they feel and how their bodies function. These techniques, autogenic training, biofeedback and physical exercise, all properly belong in the field of biogenics. It seems obvious that most patients, if they will follow the program, can gain relief from pain as well as from most psychophysiological symptoms.

CHAPTER X

Biogenic Health Maintenance

Chronic pain of a non-cancerous origin, as one of society's most devastating symptoms, has served as the focus of this book. In every instance evaluated, this symptom has been found to account for a majority of workman's compensation expenditures. Treatment of chronic pain has been exceedingly inadequate until the past few years. About eight years ago Fordyce initiated a program of operant conditioning or behavioral modification coupled with drug withdrawal as the only treatment of chronic pain patients. Over his first five years, he treated one hundred patients with 60 percent of patients improved after an eight-week, in-hospital program.

Drawing from Fordyce's experience, we organized in 1971 a pain control program which incorporated his techniques, with the addition of physiologic therapy. In about one thousand patients treated in the first two and a half years, 80 percent of them improved in the following ways:

1. Withdrawal from drugs.
2. Increased physical activity.

3. Improved emotional well-being.
4. Reduction of pain by 50 to 100 percent.

Only about 20 percent of patients achieved total pain relief during hospitalization averaging four weeks; but at least 30 percent continued to improve over the next six months. Patients continuing to improve reported that they have done so through continuing use of the mental and physical exercises taught them during therapy.

The annual cost of maintaining the disabled chronic pain patient is between five and ten thousand dollars. At the Seattle Clinic, where the cost of treatment up to 1971 averaged $5,000 per patient, Fordyce estimated that a "salvage rate" of only 10 percent justified the cost of his program. The total cost of the more comprehensive, inpatient program in LaCrosse averaged $3,400 per patient, in a non-metropolitan setting.

The physiologic therapy employed in LaCrosse includes:

1. ˙Progressive exercise (including swimming)
2. Massage
3. Heat and cold
4. Acupuncture
5. External electrical stimulation
6. Counseling
7. Autogenic training
8. Biofeedback

The last two modalities have been the major influences allowing maintenance of and continuing improvement after discharge, although all of these approaches assist in increasing activity essential to rehabilitation.

In August 1974, we converted the entire program to an intense outpatient training session of twelve days. This has allowed continuation of all the therapy except swimnastics which have been too time-consuming to allow inclusion in the twelve-day program. About 60 percent of the patient's time is spent in biofeedback and autogenic training. This entire program— biofeedback, autogenic training and physical exercise—has been called biogenics.

Autogenic training and biofeedback have also been increasingly reported successful in treatment of many psychophysiologic disturbances. Schultz, Luthe, and Green have emphasized that 80 percent of patients with a variety of psychophysiologic illnesses improve with therapy. The greatest significance of their work is the total absence of complications or iatrogenic aggravations.

These considerations lead us to suggest that health might be restored and maintained in 80 percent of patients by a comprehensive physiologic approach without the need for drugs or surgery in those problems affecting 80 percent of the population. Since a survey at one general hospital indicated that almost 60 percent of patients did not need hospitalization, but were there for convenience (or to satisfy third-party insurance requirements), the potential financial benefits seem capable of approaching the health benefits, at least quantitatively.

Restoration and maintenance of health requires a variety of approaches which integrate the complex relationship between physical and emotional stress; for all stress ultimately manifests itself in some upset of autonomic nervous system functions. Indeed, it is this loss of homeostasis which leads to most disease states. Except with trauma, infections, and congenital disorders, most illness begins with a physiological disturbance (electrical and/or chemical) manifested in the autonomic nervous system. When the stress continues, physical alterations begin. Thus, an individual may feel epigastric discomfort for a considerable time before a peptic ulcer can be identified on an X-ray.

It has been repeatedly reported by many authors that 80 to 85 percent of *symptoms* are psychosomatic; but, unfortunately, remarkably little psychophysiological therapy has been used. A number of facts indicate the need to re-orient our medical priorities. Up to 25 percent of all hospitalizations are stated to be due to iatrogenic problems. Each year 100,000 Americans are hospitalized for treatment of drug-related complications; and a large number of hospitalized patients have their confinement prolonged because of complications. Thirty thousand Americans are officially reported to die because of drug complications. Since drugs are not capable of balancing a psychophysiologic disturbance but merely attacking the predominant symptom, a more physiologic approach offers attractive alternatives.

The organization of a physiologic health center requires careful attention to diagnosis. Actually, it is in the diagnostic arena that allopathic medicine has been most successful. It is essential that proper diagnosis has excluded the need for surgery or drugs. Once diagnosis of a physiologic disturbance, or an otherwise untreatable one, has been made, patients might enter a physiologic health center in a variety of ways. These would include review by an internist or family practitioner to be certain of the diagnosis and to supervise any other diseases which require monitoring. Patients might then enter therapy in several manners:

1. Ambulatory:
   a. Unimodal therapy: patients might come in for acupuncture, external electrical stimulation instruction and therapy, autogenic training, or biofeedback.
   b. Multimodal therapy: patients enter a comprehensive day-care program using all the modalities useful for their particular problems.
2. Live in: Patients enter a minimal care facility for dormitory maintenance while involved in a multimodal program.
   a. Patients who live too far from the center for daily commuting and use the inpatient program primarily as a motel.
   b. Patients with special problems—drug withdrawal. Patients on large doses of narcotics and/or tranquilizers may require inpatient care to assure safety and proper control.

Requirements for Therapy Center:

1. Appropriate bed and dining capacity near the actual therapy.
2. Availability of consultants in most specialties.
3. Offices for professional and administrative staff.
4. Outpatient facilities.

5. *Therapy* requirements:
   a. Nurse's station
   b. Electronic device room (repairs and storage)
   c. Examining rooms—also used for interviews, acupuncture, etc.
   d. Biofeedback cubicles
   e. Cubicles for various therapies—ice, heat, massage, electrical stimulation.
   f. Exercise space
   g. Swimming pool—with built-in whirlpool
   h. Lounge (also useful for autogenic training)
   i. Laboratory—for basic tests

Illnesses which usually begin as physiological disturbances are:

1. Migraine
2. Atherosclerosis
3. Benign hypertension
4. Peptic ulcers
5. Impotentia
6. Tension, anxiety, and most behavioral disorders
7. Spastic colon and chronic constipation
8. Dizziness
9. Neurodermatitis
10. Disorders of immunity which *probably* include: multiple sclerosis, ALS, scleroderma, lupus erythematosus, rheumatoid arthritis, cancer, and most metabolic disorders.

In many other illnesses, physiologic abnormalities contribute to continuing symptoms or disability.

1. Back and neck injuries
2. Cerebral palsy
3. Post surgical symptoms
4. Chronic pain states

All of these symptoms and syndromes are part of the "Games People Play." Many are included in the "Pain Game." Biogenics has been designed to help physicians and patients play this game to a satisfactory solution.

Diseases which are not amenable to treatment in such a center:

1. Most acute problems, including trauma, heart attacks, congestive heart failure, infections, GI bleeding, cerebral hemorrhage, pulmonary embolus.
2. Those problems requiring surgery (but post-op recovery may be handled).
3. Liver or kidney failure or other terminal diseases.
4. Cancer (initially). After appropriate initial treatment, autogenics may be useful.
5. Psychoses—the remarkably different therapy required in these problems suggests the need for development of alternative health care facilities and programs for them.

In order to accomplish these goals, *true* health maintenance organizations using a biogenic foundation need to be developed. Ideally patients desiring the best possible health and wishing to practice prevention of disease would contract for a thorough course in biogenics. They would learn the best diet, and mental and physical exercises. Trace mineral analyses would be done and proper balance effected. Refresher courses in biogenics could be taken electively at any time. The total professional personnel required would be far less than in disease-oriented medical systems. Such a health program could be a total, comprehensive prepaid health system. I believe it could be delivered to the American people at a cost which is at least no greater than current medical cost but at a quality which is quite superior. It would almost certainly eliminate *at least half* the hospitalizations and surgeries done in traditional systems and probably 80 percent or more of drugs. These accomplishments in themselves are almost guarantees of better health!

APPENDIX

PAIN QUESTIONNAIRE

This booklet contains a series of questions designed to help your physician evaluate and treat your pain. The answers are confidential and of use only to your physician.

Please do not write in this booklet. Use the answer sheet supplied and select the proper set of lines for each question. Most questions should have only one best answer. There is no right or wrong answer; choose the answer which fits *you.* Do not skip any questions.

Be sure the number of the statement agrees with the number on the answer sheet. Make your marks heavy and black. Erase completely any answers you wish to change.

Do not make *any* marks in this booklet. Try to mark an answer to each question on the answer sheet.

Sample section of answer sheet correctly marked:

This year is
   a. before 1970   1. a. =
   b. after 1970   b. ▬

Considerable assistance in preparing this questionnaire has been received from Dr. Ron Melzack, Professor of Psychology, McGill University, Montreal.

This booklet has been designed for patients with chronic pain. Individual answers will be available to your physician for comparison with his other patients. Each patient's answers are confidential. Prepared as a service to physicians by THE PAIN REHABILITATION CENTER, 615 South 10th Street, La Crosse, Wisconsin 54601.

1. Age
   a. less than 30
   b. 30-45
   c. 45-60
   d. over 60

2. Education
   a. grade school
   b. high school
   c. college
   d. masters
   e. doctorate

3. Your best income
   a. less than $10,000 annually
   b. $10-20,000 annually
   c. over $20,000 annually

4. Marital situation
   a. married once
   b. married more than once
   c. divorced
   d. single
   e. widowed

5. Occupation
   a. housewife
   b. desk job
   c. driving car, bus, or truck
   d. walking a lot
   e. heavy work
   f. professional

6. Religion
   a. Catholic
   b. Protestant
   c. Jewish
   d. Other organized religion
   e. Atheist

7. Previous psychiatric evaluation?
   a. yes
   b. no

8. Previous psychiatric treatment for greater than 1 month?
   a. yes
   b. no

9. Chiropractic adjustments?
   a. yes
   b. no

10. Has psychiatric treatment been suggested?
    a. yes
    b. no

11. Have you ever desired it?
    a. yes
    b. no

12. I feel that psychiatric help is
    a. excellent
    b. occasionally good
    c. a waste of time and money

13. Your leisure time activities before onset of pain:
    a. sedentary (bridge, etc.)
    b. moderate activity (gardening, etc.)
    c. vigorous sports

14. Your leisure activities now:
    a. sedentary (bridge, etc.)
    b. moderate activity (gardening, etc.)
    c. vigorous sports

15. Length of time you've had pain
    a. less than 1 year
    b. less than 2 years
    c. less than 5 years
    d. less than 10 years
    e. over 10 years

16. Describe your personality
    a. tense
    b. anxious
    c. cool, well-adjusted
    d. nervous
    e. excitable
    f. happy
    g. depressed

17. Your intellectual ability
    a. average
    b. below average
    c. above average

18. Your physical health other than related to pain
    a. excellent
    b. good
    c. fair
    d. poor

19. Your financial support now:
   a. husband or wife working
   b. self supporting
   c. workmen's compensation payments
   d. disability insurance
   e. social security
   f. personal investments or income

Wife or Husband

20. Age
   a. less than 30
   b. 30-45
   c. 45-60
   d. over 60

21. Education
   a. grade school
   b. high school
   c. college
   d. masters
   e. doctorate

22. Occupation
   a. housewife
   b. desk job
   c. driving job
   d. walking job
   e. heavy work
   f. professional

23. Leisure time activities before onset of pain
   a. sedentary (bridge, etc.)
   b. moderate activity (gardening, etc.)
   c. vigorous sports

24. Leisure activities now
   a. sedentary (bridge, etc.)
   b. moderate activity (gardening, etc.)
   c. vigorous sports

25. Describe his or her personality
   a. tense
   b. anxious
   c. depressed
   d. cool, well-adjusted
   e. nervous
   f. excitable
   g. happy

26. Your relationship with spouse
   a. excellent
   b. average
   c. poor

Father

27. Age
   a. 30-45
   b. 45-60
   c. over 60
   d. deceased

28. Education
   a. grade school
   b. high school
   c. college
   d. masters
   e. doctorate

29. Occupation
   a. desk job
   b. driving job
   c. walking job
   d. heavy work
   e. professional

30. Leisure time activities
   a. sedentary (bridge, etc.)
   b. moderate activity (gardening, etc.)
   c. vigorous sports

31. Describe his personality
   a. tense
   b. anxious
   c. depressed
   d. cool, well-adjusted
   e. nervous
   f. excitable
   g. happy

32. Your relation with him
   a. excellent
   b. average
   c. poor

Mother

33. Age
   a. 30-45
   b. 45-60
   c. over 60
   d. deceased

34. Education
   a. grade school
   b. high school
   c. college
   d. masters
   e. doctorate

35. Occupation
   a. housewife
   b. desk job
   c. driving job
   d. walking job
   e. heavy work
   f. professional

36. Leisure time acitivites
   a. sedentary (bridge, etc.)
   b. moderate activity (gardening, etc.)
   c. vigorous sports

37. Describe her personality
   a. tense
   b. anxious
   c. depressed
   d. cool, well-adjusted
   e. nervous
   f. excitable
   g. happy

38. Your relation with her
   a. excellent
   b. average
   c. poor

Siblings (brothers and sisters)

39. Number
    a. one
    b. two
    c. more than two
    d. none

40. Your relationship with siblings
    a. excellent
    b. average
    c. poor

Your Children

41. Number
    a. one
    b. two
    c. more than two
    d. none

42. Your relationship with your children
    a. excellent
    b. average
    c. poor

(PLEASE ANSWER QUESTIONS 43 THROUGH 93 ABOUT YOURSELF AND YOUR PAIN)

43. Cause of pain
    a. accident
    b. doctor
    c. previous treatment or surgery
    d. scar
    e. nature

44. Surgeries done to correct problem
    a. laminectomy once
    b. laminectomy twice
    c. laminectomy three times or more
    d. laminectomy with fusion
    e. amputation
    f. freeing of scar
    g. removal of tumor
    h. other

45. Surgeries done just to relieve pain
    a. sympathectomy
    b. rhizotomy
    c. cordotomy, surgical
    d. cordotomy by needle
    e. cingulumotomy
    f. other

46. When does pain occur?
    a. at rest
    b. sitting
    c. walking
    d. with working or lifting
    e. all the time
    f. less than 8 hours/day
    g. 8-16 hours/day
    h. during sexual intercourse

47. How long do you have to rest to relieve pain once is starts?
   a. less than 30 minutes
   b. at least one hour
   c. several hours or more

48. What relieves pain?
   a. sex
   b. lying
   c. sitting
   d. drugs
   e. heat
   f. massage
   g. traction
   h. other

49. Use of alcohol
   a. none
   b. moderate
   c. heavy

50. Use of cigarettes
   a. none
   b. less than 1 pack/day
   c. about 1 pack/day
   d. 2 or more packs/day

51. How many hours in a day are you free of pain?
   a. less than 8
   b. 8-16
   c. 16-24

52. How many hours do you lie down in each 24?
   a. less than 8
   b. 8-12
   c. 12-16
   d. 16-18
   e. 18-24

53. Would you work if you had no pain?
   a. yes
   b. no
   c. full time
   d. part time

54. Do you have difficulty having sexual intercourse?
   a. yes
   b. no

55. How many times do you have sexual intercourse each month?
   a. 0-1
   b. 2
   c. 3
   d. 4-7
   e. 8 or more

56. Does pain interfere with sexual intercourse?
   a. yes
   b. no

57. Does sexual stimulation mask your pain?
   a. yes
   b. no

58. What kind of mattress do you have?

   a. hard
   b. soft
   c. innerspring
   d. foam rubber

59. Do you have a compensation claim or law suit pending?

   a. yes
   b. no

60. What result do you expect from us?

   a. nothing
   b. complete pain relief
   c. ability to return to work
   d. partial pain relief

61. Where is your pain?

   a. head
   b. neck
   c. right arm
   d. left arm
   e. chest
   f. abdomen
   g. pelvis, groin, rectum
   h. right leg
   i. left leg
   j. back

We are indebted to Melzack & Torgerson, "On The Language of Pain," *Anesthesiology*, 1971, 34:50-59, for questions 62-90.

What Does Your Pain Feel Like?

Some of the words below describe your present pain. Select ONLY those words that best describe it. Use only a single word in each appropriate category — the one that applies best.

62.
   a. flickering
   b. quivering
   c. pulsing
   d. throbbing
   e. beating
   f. pounding
   g. none of these

63.
   a. jumping
   b. flashing
   c. shooting
   d. none of these

64.
   a. pricking
   b. boring
   c. drilling
   d. stabbing
   e. lancinating
   f. none of these

65.
   a. sharp
   b. cutting
   c. lacerating
   d. none of these

66.
   a. pinching
   b. pressing
   c. gnawing
   d. cramping
   e. crushing
   f. none of these

67.
   a. tugging
   b. pulling
   c. wrenching
   d. none of these

68.
a. hot
b. burning
c. scalding
d. searing
e. none of these

69.
a. tingling
b. itchy
c. smarting
d. stinging
e. none of these

70.
a. dull
b. sore
c. hurting
d. aching
e. heavy
f. none of these

71.
a. tender
b. taut
c. rasping
d. splitting
e. none of these

72.
a. tiring
b. exhausting
c. none of these

73.
a. sickening
b. suffocating
c. none of these

74.
a. fearful
b. frightful
c. terrifying
d. none of these

75.
a. punishing
b. gruelling
c. cruel
d. vicious
e. killing
f. none of these

76.
a. wretched
b. blinding
c. none of these

77.
a. annoying
b. troublesome
c. miserable
d. intense
e. unbearable
f. none of these

78.
a. spreading
b. radiating
c. penetrating
d. piercing
e. none of these

79.
a. tight
b. numb
c. drawing
d. squeezing
e. tearing
f. none of these

80.
a. cool
b. cold
c. freezing
d. none of these

81.
a. nagging
b. nauseating
c. agonizing
d. dreadful
e. torturing
f. none of these

How Does Your Pain Change With Time?

Which word or words would you use to describe the *pattern* of your pain.

82.
a. continuous
b. steady
c. constant
d. none of these

83.
a. rhythmic
b. periodic
c. intermittent
d. none of these

84.
a. brief
b. momentary
c. transient
d. none of these

How Strong Is Your Pain?

People agree that the following 5 words represent pain of increasing intensity. They are:

    a. mild
    b. discomforting
    c. distressing
    d. horrible
    e. excruciating

To answer each question below, fill in your answer on the answer sheet using the most appropriate word from above.

85. Which word describes your pain right now?

86. Which word describes it at its worst?

87. Which word describes it when it is least?

88. Which word describes the worst toothache you ever had?

89. Which word describes the worst headache you ever had?

90. Which word describes the worst stomach ache you ever had?

91. Your work history:

    a. same job over 5 years
    b. more than 2 jobs in past 5 years
    c. no work for 1 year
    d. no work for over 2 years
    e. retired because of age

Your Present Medications

92. Pain relievers
    a. Aspirin
    b. Talwin shots
    c. Talwin pills
    d. Darvon
    e. Demerol
    f. Percodan
    g. Codeine
    h. Methadon
    i. Other narcotics

93. Other drugs
    a. Thorazine
    b. Elavil
    c. Tofranil
    d. Soma
    e. Valium
    f. Phenergan
    g. Librium
    h. Barbiturates
    i. Dilantin
    j. Others

BIBLIOGRAPHY

Beals, Rodney K., and Norman W. Hickman, "Industrial injuries of the back and extremities," *Journal of Bone and Joint Surgery,* **54:** 1593, 1972.

Bolen, Jean Shinoda, "Meditation and psychotherapy in the treatment of cancer," *Psychic,* **19,** July/August, 1973.

Chao, Y., et. al., "A new method of preventing adhesions: the use of aminoplastic after craniotomy," *British Medical Journal,* **1:** 517, 1940.

Cloward, R.B., "Cervical discography: a contribution to the etiology and mechanism of neck, shoulder, and arm pain," *Annals of Surgery,* **150:** 1052, 1959.

Fowler, Raymond, *The MMPI Notebook.* Roche Psychiatric Service Institute, 1966

Freese, Arthur S., *Headaches.* New York: Doubleday, 1973.

Freese, Arthur S., *Pain.* New York: Putnam, 1974.

Gentry, W. Doyle, W. Derek Shows, and Michael Thomas, "Chronic low back pain: a psychological profile," *Psychosomatic Medicine,* **XV:** 174, 1974.

Gladman, Arthur E., and Norma Estrada, "Preliminary observations on the clinical application of biofeedback." Unpublished paper.

Hitselberger, W.E., and R.N. Witten, "Abnormal myelograms in asymptomatic patients," *Journal of Neurosurgery,* **28:** 204, 1968.

Hosobuchi, J., J.E. Adams, and P.R. Weinstein, "Preliminary percutaneous dorsal column stimulation prior to permanent inplantation (technical note)," *Journal of Neurosurgery,* **37:** 242, 1972.

Hymes, Alan C., D.E. Raab, E.G. Yonehira, G.D. Nelson, and A.L. Printy, "Acute pain control by electrostimulation: a preliminary report," *Advances in Neurological Sciences,* **4:** 761, 1974.

Kamimura, M., and T. Matsuzawa, "Free dermal fat grafting," *Japanese Journal of Plastic and Reconstructive Surgery,* **8:** 150, 1965.

Kellaway, P., "The William Oster medal essay — the part played by electric fish in the early history of bioelectricity and electrotherapy," *Bulletin of the History of Medicine,* **20:** 112, 1946.

Larson, J., A. Sances, Jr., D.H. Reigel, and D. Dallman, "Application of current to the spinal cord." Paper presented at the Third International Symposium on Electrosleep and electroanesthesia, Varna, Bulgaria, 1972.

Lintilhac, J.P., et al, "Dulopillo's dressing: the role of prolonged continuous elastic compression in the prevention of retractile and hypertrophic scars, *Maroc-Medical,* **45:** 253, 1966.

Mayfield, F.H., and M.S. O'Brien, "Postoperative segmental adhesive arachnoiditis (or pachymeningitis): a method of surgical treatment." Paper presented to the Harvey Cushing Society, St. Louis, Missouri, April 20 1966.

Melzack, Ronald, *The Puzzle of Pain.* New York: Basic Books, 1974.

Melzack, R., and P.D. Wall, "Pain mechanisms: a new theory," *Science,* **150:** 971, 1965.

Mixter, W.J., and J.S. Barr, "Rupture of the intervertebral disc with involvement of the spinal canal," *New England Journal of Medicine,* **211:** 210, 193ᵃ

Peacock, E.E., "Inter- and intramolecular bonding in collagen of healing wounds by insertion of methylene and amide cross-links into scar tissue: tensile strength and thermal shrinkage in rats," *Annals of Surgery,* **163:** 1, 1966.

Richards D.E., J.S. Brodkey, and F.E. Nulson, "A mechanism for pain inhibition by dorsal column stimulation." Paper presented to the American Association of Neurological Surgeons, April, 1972.

Shapiro, David, Bernard Tursky, Elliot Gershon, and Melvin Stern, "Effects of feedback and reinforcement on the control of human systolic blood pressure," *Science,* **163:** 588, 1969.

Sargent, Joseph D., Elmer E. Green, and Dale E. Walters, "The use of autogenic feedback training in a pilot study of migraine and tension headaches," *Headache,* **12:** 120, 1972.

Timmermans, Gretchen, and Richard A. Sternbach, "Factors of human chronic pain: an analysis of personality and pain reaction variables," *Science,* **184:** 806, 1974.

White, J.C., "Results in surgical treatment of herniated lumbar intervertebral discs: investigation of the late results in subject with and without supplementary spinal fusion—a preliminary report," *Clinical Neurology,* **13:** 42, 1966.

Wickramasekira, Ian, "Electromyographic feedback training and tension headache: preliminary observations," *American Journal of Clinical Hypnosis,* **15:** 83, 1972.

Willis, William D., Jr., "Neurophysiological basis of doral column stimulation for the relief of pain." Paper presented at a symposium in Dallas, Texas, April, 1971.

INDEX

143

BOOKS OF RELATED INTEREST

THE HEALING MIND, the controversial, disturbing, fascinating first book by noted lecturer and medical researcher Dr. Irving Oyle, describes what is known about the mysterious ability of the mind to heal the body. 128 pages, soft cover, $4.95

MAGIC, MYSTICISM AND MODERN MEDICINE by Dr. Irving Oyle offers fascinating glimpses into the lives and minds of many who came to the doctor's experimental community health service and the new methods of healing he was compelled to explore. 128 pages, soft cover, $4.95

In **TIME, SPACE AND THE MIND,** Dr. Irving Oyle examines the mind's ability to switch off time/space reality and produce the single most powerful healing tool available to humanity. Dr. Oyle draws on his 20 years of experience as a family physician. 160 pages, soft cover, $4.95

Stanley Krippner and Alberto Villoldo's **REALMS OF HEALING** presents a scientific exploration of non-medical healing and healers around the world, with emphasis on current laboratory research in the United States, the USSR, Brazil and Canada. 252 pages, soft cover, $7.95

WHOLLY ALIVE by Drs. Barry Saltzman, Richard Kaplan and Lawrence Ecker, with Patrick Wilkins, is the holistic doctors' health book and explains how we all can be wholly - to the fullest extent - alive. Not just partially well but in the best of health in body and mind. 160 pages, soft cover, $4.95

Available at your local book or department store or directly from the publisher. To order by mail, send check or money order to:

Celestial Arts
231 Adrian Road
Millbrae, Ca. 94030

Please add $1.00 for postage and handling. California residents add 6% tax.